BREAD
IN THE
MODERN DIET

BREAD
IN THE
MODERN
DIET
KELLY GREGG MD

TABLE OF CONTENTS

Introduction

This book continues the journey of diet and health. Something has happened to our diet so that now obesity, type 2 diabetes, cancer, and autoimmune disease has greatly increased in incidence and prevalence in the last generation or so. I have zeroed in on insulin resistance as the common driving force for many of these problems. In the beginning, I presented the disease of diabetes, and how it evolves from insulin resistance. A step back showed obesity to be a precursor. A step back revealed diet to be the main driver. I then went through the elements of the diet that have changed over the last five thousand years and how these changes have led to our current state.

It ends up that the processing of foods may be leading the way toward our current state. I felt obligated to at least put out the fire and discussed the ketogenic diet as the most effective fat-loss diet (other than fasting). This is a temporary diet, and unless you change what you eat, you end up back at the same place. What was needed is a guideline as to how someone could construct a diet to be used for a lifetime, that would increase the chances for health. Carbohydrates play the starring role in insulin resistance. Sucrose (and high fructose corn syrup) have become the processed foods that are leading the way as far as insulin resistance; but most of our glucose comes from starch, and that main starch ends up being bread, the first processed food in human history. Since we have been eating bread since the beginning, why is it now causing us a problem?

This book is a continuation of the previous book, *Maintenance Diet for the Modern Man*. Bread has been such a vital part of the history of man's diet that it required its own book to adequately show its relationship to insulin resistance.

Your diet is what you eat, when you eat, when you don't eat, and how you absorb what you eat. Thus far, I have concentrated on glucose and subsequent insulin resistance, but the gut microbiome may turn out to be equally important, as is the growing of modern food, the processing of modern food, and the chemicals in modern food (and environment). These may be playing an equal role; not only in modern disease but also in your fundamental genetic makeup and expression.

BREAD

Before we start, this book is a continuation of my last book, *Maintenance Diet for the Modern Man,* which is the last book in a tetralogy about diet and health. These books were born of the observation that over the last generation or so, man seems to be experiencing a higher standard of living, but decreased health: that being the ability to work, function, enjoy life, and be content. The incidence of obesity, prediabetes, and diabetes is now over 40% in the United States and rising throughout the western world, along with the incidence of cancer and autoimmune disease. Although there may be several elements in our modern life contributing to this epidemic, diet is by far the largest factor associated with obesity and type 2 diabetes, and one that we can control. The first book, *Diabetes, Prediabetes, Obesity: Management, Prevention, Treatment,* examined the principal dietary disease and how it develops from what we eat. The next, *The Ketogenic Diet for Beginners,* discussed the metabolic basis for what I consider to be the best fat-loss diet. The next, *Autophagy for the Common Man*, discusses a process in humans that enables cellular replacement and maintains health, and may be a large part of the benefits of fasting. The last, *Maintenance Diet,* is the diet you pursue when you have reached a stable state after losing weight.

This diet for a normal person is not the same as it is for someone who has prediabetes. It is a guidebook for the food engineer, the person who buys the food, prepares the food, and serves the food. This person must design and prepare a diet for infants, teenagers, adults, and the elderly; providing enough calories, develop tasty meals, and making nutritious foods that prevent the development of obesity and other nutritional diseases. It is a guidebook for a 30-year diet.

I have based much of my research on diet by comparing the diet of man in the previous 5000 years, with the diet in the last 200 years. The Bible provides historical context as does the Egyptian world empire, as well as providing written records. Over most of the last few thousand years, there has not been much famine (unless related to government interventions), nor much obesity. Of course, this is a biased history as without a reliable food supply you could not have much of a civilization, hence no written records. Most of the dietary pathology has occurred just in the last 70 years, within my lifetime and experience. Nowadays, most recognize that what these diseases have in common is insulin resistance. My previous books review this subject and its etiology, as well as the treatment.

The result of studying dietary history left me with a conundrum. Grains have been used from the beginning, as both a source of food and one of the primary ways food was stored to avoid starvation during seasons of food scarcity. In almost every western civilization it accounted for the bulk of caloric intake, around 50% of the diet, and often more. At the same time, the treatment for obesity is to lower carbohydrate ingestion. If bread is mainly carbohydrates, why didn't we get insulin resistance in historical societies?

Is there something different about bread made 3000 years ago as opposed to bread made 300 years ago? The answer is yes. You can see that in the images of bread over the years. Bread was described and depicted as a firm, brown loaf that was fairly flat. It staled rapidly and there are many recipes for leftover stale bread. Now we have light white bread, soft crusts, and it lasts for a few weeks. It is not surprising that this has occurred, as most people want this type of bread. With the development of capitalism in certain countries, the millers competed to make flour that would result in this type of bread to make more money. The bakers have also changed the way they used this flour, along with the usage of additives. This has continued to the present day and we now have white, light, fluffy bread wherever bread is sold. Sliced bread has only been around about one hundred years.

The goal of the *Maintenance Diet* book was to provide a basis for a lifelong diet for the family, both young and old, that would be practical, and the basis for maintaining good health. To do that, I went through the biochemistry and metabolism to establish a basis for a healthy diet, as well as the reasons the current American diet was leading to obesity. I did not give any recipes, but just general principles. When I was faced with incorporating bread into this diet, it became evident that this was a major topic, so large that I could not include it within the last book without surpassing the economic length of an Amazon book.

I therefore have written this book on bread, almost as an addendum to the last book. Therefore, I will not include my normal chapters on biochemistry and metabolism. That's not to say I will not provide information on the science of bread making, but you will have to read another book if you want the complete package of what happens when you eat and don't eat. This book is an informational book and guideline for the use of bread and grains in the maintenance diet. It is not a cookbook, but in the end, you will understand the ingredients in bread and how to adapt them to your family's diet.

Bread is composed of flour, liquid (water), salt, and yeast. This is true for leavened bread, which is bread whose dough can expand as a result of CO_2 production by the yeast. For this to occur, the flour must contain the proteins of gluten, which form an elastic framework to trap the gas. The grains that contain gluten are those from wheat, rye, and barley: these have been the primary grains to make flour in the history of western civilization and I will confine my discussion of bread to these grains (a note about oats later). Rye and Barley are also gluten-containing grains and, although they were also a good source of carbohydrates and protein in history, wheat still was the dominant source. The bread is also baked, which gives the dough some time to rise before setting the dough and crust.

There are probably thousands of different recipes for this type of bread, but the principles of nutrition are similar for all. In some form, bread is usually a part of the modern diet. Historically it served as a primary source of protein, fat, and carbohydrates and has prevented starvation throughout the world. In modern times bread is fortified with vitamins and minerals that were removed by modern milling, but before that time, bread was a necessary part of the diet to maintain health. There are many different flatbreads made with different ingredients that do not contain gluten, but I will confine my discussion to the normal bread loaf you buy at the store.

GRAIN

Bread starts with flour, and flour starts with grain. Wheat is the oldest domesticated crop and numerous varieties have been developed over the last few thousand years. This occurs through cross-fertilization and there is no GMO wheat. Although there are no GMO varieties, that does not keep seed companies from deliberately exposing grains to mutagens, such as radiation or some chemicals, to try to induce a useful mutation. The simplest wheat contains one pair of seven chromosomes, so each cell contains 14 chromosomes. Although humans have 23 pairs of chromosomes for a total of 46 in each cell, wheat chromosomes are much larger, and one pair has ten times the number of genes as a pair of human chromosomes. This is even more complicated as wheat cells can contain two sets of paired chromosomes (a total of 28 chromosomes) and almost all bread wheat now contains three sets of paired chromosomes (total of 42 chromosomes). This is one reason there are 30,000 to 50,000 different varieties of wheat. In the US, we use about 500-1000 varieties to make bread flour. You can see how versatile this plant can be as different varieties can be planted depending on the climate (hot, warm, or cool), the rainfall, the type of soil, the plant disease in that region, the amount of protein desired or even the time to maturation. This is one reason that so much wheat is cultivated as it is adaptable to conditions and altitudes all over the world.

I am writing this book for the food engineer. A few may be motivated to grind their own wheat, but most will just buy flour or just buy bread; even so, knowledge of grain and flour will help you choose the best diet for your family. So far, I have only spoken about wheat. Rye and barley were used for breadmaking for thousands of years and still today, but wheat has taken over the modern diet and these other grains are just niche breads. That's not to say they can contribute to a varied and flavorful diet, and I would encourage the food engineer to incorporate these breads in the diet. First, what is grain?

Grain is just a small, hard, dry seed. A cereal grain is one derived from a grass plant and contains the outer bran, the fat and protein-containing germ, and the starch-containing endosperm. This starch consists of starch granules that are individually trapped in a protein matrix which contains various proteins, including the ones that form gluten. When you remove the bran and germ, you still retain about 75% of the wheat protein and 83% of the weight of the kernels. The fat is mainly contained in the germ, which is why it was removed for hundreds of years to increase the flour shelf life, as the fat undergoes oxidation and spoils the taste of the bread. Now we add chemicals to preserve the flour which extends the shelf life to at least 9 months. In a dry climate the grain can last over a year. Before chemicals, you needed to save the food you harvested for about a year before you harvested again. This conveniently supplied you with food over the winter.

If you got it milled into flour, you decreased the shelf life quite a bit. If you removed the germ, you extend this shelf life. If your local water mill could only run part of the year (if the water froze, the mill stopped) or if you could only get to the mill when the weather allowed travel, you couldn't always mill the grain just when you needed it and had to figure out how to store flour. These problems have mainly existed for the last 700 years. Before that time, you would store the grain in a dry place at home, and just grind the grain at home when you needed it. With the advancement of technology, nobody does this anymore (except maybe the people reading this book).

I believe almost everyone agrees that whole grains provide more nutrition than white flour. Why then would anyone eat white bread. For most of mankind's history, we ate whole wheat. It was difficult not to use this type of flour as hand or stone milling is not amenable to routine removal of bran and germ. This bread was darker, heavier, and denser than modern bread and, it also staled more rapidly. When large scale milling became popular, we could separate the bran and the germ from the grain by a judicious shifting of the flour. This allowed the millers to make a finer flour that was lighter and less dense. People wanted this type of bread. Eventually, we figured out what vitamins and minerals were so that about 80 years ago we began adding these back to the flour (enriched). We didn't go back to whole wheat because, no matter how you make it, whole wheat flour makes darker, denser bread than modern white flour, and now people were accustomed to light, fluffy bread. You can buy whole wheat bread at the store, but if you look at the ingredients, you see we must add a lot to make it look like modern bread.

I am going to have to recommend the modern food engineer use whole wheat flour, just like we did for thousands of years. You could grind your own, but in the last 20 years, there has been enough information about nutrition available that the capitalistic system is working and whole wheat flour is available wherever you shop. I am also going to have to recommend organic flour. Maximum wheat production often involves the use of chemicals to fight molds, bacteria, pests, and viruses, and I don't recommend a steady diet of these chemicals. Remember, whole wheat flour brings us back to the problem of storage as now we have the germ again, therefore, store these in a cool, dry place in air-tight containers if possible. When whole wheat flour is milled with a roller mill, the bran and germ are separated from endosperm, the endosperm is milled, and the bran and germ are added back later. With stone ground flour, the whole grain is used and not separated. The particle size is going to be larger, and it is going to be more difficult to make fluffy bread. As you will read later, roller milling flour particles to a small size may induce insulin resistance.

I am going to recommend organic, stone-ground, whole-wheat flour. It may be necessary to occasionally use white flour as some items just won't work well with whole wheat (cakes, biscuits); but for the most part, use whole wheat. This will make more sense later in the book.

Back to the types of wheat grain. Virtually all flour we use is from bread wheat, which contains three sets of chromosomes. When you buy flour, you are getting all kinds of different varieties (500-1000) that are used to make flour, depending on what part of the country, or even which part of the state grew the grain. I will give you a little info about historical flour. You could go online and buy flour made from any of these grains, or even buy the whole grain.

We will initially separate the types of grains into hulled grain and non-hulled. The hull is a strong covering of the grain which protects the grain from the environment and insects. These look like small berries. When hulled wheat is thrashed, you end up with a tough covering of the grain that requires some type of processing to remove the husk. You then have the grain which can be processed in the usual way. In free-thrashing wheat, there is no hull and the grain is easily removed for milling.

Einhorn is a diploid wheat (one set of seven chromosomes {14}) and was grown early in history. It is hulled. You can buy Einhorn grain or flour, but it is rarely used.

Emmer is a tetraploid wheat (two sets of seven chromosomes {28}) and was also grown early on. It is hulled. You can buy Emmer grain or flour. It is rarely used now a days.

Spelt is a hexaploidy wheat (three sets of seven chromosomes {42} and was popular later in history. It is hulled. You can buy this grain or flour and is more popular than the others listed.

Remember there are many varieties of each of these. They all contain gluten. Their baking properties are slightly different from the modern bread wheat.

The Egyptians in the Nile valley were prolific growers of wheat for about the last 5000 years, even to this present day. This was the basis for their world empire as civilization cannot exist without an excess of food. The wheat grown through much of this period was Emmer. This is hulled wheat, so it had to be harvested, processed to remove the hulls, winnowed to separate the hulls from the grain, and then the grain made into flour. During the seven years of great famine, the wheat stored in the granaries from the previous seven years of plenty was Emmer. A hulled wheat like Emmer stored in a dry climate would easily last the seven years of famine. The most common food was bread, the most common drink in Egypt at this time was beer, made from Emmer wheat; hence the brewing process provided a source of yeast for non-sourdough bread.

Durum is a tetraploid wheat that is free-thrashing (no hull) and widely used today. It as a high percentage of protein (gluten) and is used in pasta and macaroni as the dough is plastic and can be easily formed. It is the second most common grain used next to common (bread) wheat. Durum is milled to a coarse size called semolina. There is a fine flour from durum that can be used to make bread or add to the pastas. You can buy the grain and make your own pasta, of course, you will need to mill it.

Bread wheat accounts for 95% of the flour made and there are many different varieties of grains used; we can divide these up into a few classes:

Hard Red Winter: high-protein and used for bread making. These grains can be bought in bulk at some health food stores. Hard wheat means it has a higher protein content and is probably what you are getting when you buy unbleached all-purpose flour. Winter wheat means it is planted in the fall and harvested the next summer. This is grown in the Great Plains

Hard Red spring: It is also high-protein and used for bread and baked goods. Planted in the spring and harvested in the fall. This is grown in the northern regions and Canada.

Hard White: Medium-protein and naturally light-colored. This is planted in temperate, dry climates.

Soft White: Lower protein and used for pie crusts and pastry where you don't want a lot of gluten and dough rising.

Most of the time when you buy bread at the store, your choice is white bread, whole wheat, 100% whole wheat, and stone ground. If not stated as stone-ground, it is probably roller milled, and not 100% whole wheat, and, probably not organic.

Hulled barley means the outer hull is removed. Pearled means the bran layer is also removed. So hulled would be the same as 100% whole barley.

You can apply the same definitions for Rye.

Most of you are just going to buy bread. Sometimes you will be unable to get 100% whole wheat, as when you get rolls or baguettes. At least avoid always using white, fluffy bread.

Some of you will make some of your bread products. I have given you some information which will help you to decide what kind of flour to get. Now you get a dozen different choices when you go to the store.

Few of you will make your own flour. This group knows more about breadmaking than I do. Just try to use coarser particle sizes. It will make it slightly harder to make a less dense bread, but as you will read, it may be of benefit to you.

FLOUR

Flour is a powder made by grinding roots, beans, nuts, seeds, or grains. For my purpose, I will confine the discussion to the cereal grains we just discussed. You know about the different types and classes of grain, enough that you have some idea of what you are getting when you order grains to grind yourself. The result of this grinding, or milling, is going to be flour; so, no matter if you do it yourself or buy it from the store, we end up with flour. Remember the grain is the seed of the plant and contains an embryonic plant with enough nutrition to enable the plant to produce roots and leaves prior to photosynthesis starting. Let's look at the seed.

We already know that the wheat grain is composed of three parts: bran, germ, and endosperm. The bran contains the husk and indigestible cellulose, the germ contains the protein, and the endosperm the starch. Of course, life is not that simple. The bran is not just a very thin layer over the seed but is about 15% of the weight to the grain, as opposed to the germ which is only 3%. There are three general layers of the bran covering: Aleurone layer (about 8% of the grain weight), testa layer (1%), and the pericarp layer (4%) divided into inner and outer.

The aleurone layer contains soluble and insoluble fiber, proteins and enzymes, essential amino acids, vitamin E and B, minerals (may be complexed with phytic acid, lipids, plant cholesterols. The testa layer contains sterols, alkylresorcinols, and stearyl ferulates. You can look up these compounds but essentially, they are complex molecules that can be used by your body. Pericarp contains insoluble dietary fiber and antioxidants. The point of these sentences is to get you to realize that bran is not just some cellulose cover that only serves to protect the seed from the environment. The bran is rich enough in nutrients that it can be a component of cattle fodder.

Dietary fiber is not just cellulose. It is composed of indigestible carbohydrates with various chemical structures that are resistant to the enzymes in the gut you use to break down the rest of your nutrients so that they can be absorbed. Wheat bran is about 50% dietary fiber (insoluble), about 5% soluble. Your gut biome is composed of billions of bacteria that can metabolize some of this fiber, and it is an important source of nutrients for this vital organ of your body. More on the gut biome in a different book.

Most of the flour sold has the bran removed. After reading the above, why would anyone want to do this? I am going to write a section on milling below, but before we get too hard on these people, we must recognize what type of food bread was for most of history up to the last 150 years. The bread was a hard, tough, heavy, dense food. It could be used as a container for soup or as a plate on which to eat food. After about a day, it was difficult to eat unless soaked in water or some other liquid (toasting at a speech was bread dipped in beer or wine). This was not done for show, it was just the bread was too hard to eat. I agree it was nutritious and portable and would last several days if you were traveling, but it was nothing like the bread we eat today. Many techniques were tried to make the bread more palpable, but coarse whole wheat bread dough just does not rise that well. As time went on, grain with more gluten was developed and instead of natural yeast (sourdough) or leftover brewer's yeast, some better baker's yeast was developed; it still was a heavy dense product with a tough crust. Those of you who grind and bake with your own wheat at home, despite using modern grain, know what kind of bread this is, so give these millers a break when they figured out how to make light, fluffy bread.

The first wheat was hulled. This required breaking down the hull which was performed using something like a mortar and pestle. Then the grain was winnowed to separate the husk from the grain, then the grain was ground up to produce smaller particles. For most of history, this consisted of rubbing the grain between two stones. This enables one to get to a small enough size (about ½ a millimeter or about 500 microns) to make a bread that did not feel grainy. This flour had a range of particle sizes, but as long as the largest was less than about 500 microns, the bread had a reasonable texture. When we started out, the grain did not have a lot of gluten and did not rise much with the addition of natural (sourdough) yeast, but the cultivation of wheat parallels the development of civilization and also the brewing of beer; so there was extra yeast around to use and some people did not like the sour part of sourdough bread.

The milling of wheat by the rubbing of two stones together was slowly made more efficient, till the Romans developed grist mills where this could be done in larger quantities. During this time, the bakers figured out that if you could remove the bran from the whole wheat flour, the bread would have a better texture, rise a little bit more, and be a little lighter in color; it was just not very easy to do, so the flour without as much bran was a premium product. Everybody wanted it but few could afford it. Even 3500 years ago the Mosaic law advises the offerings to be made of fine flour, indicating that even then it was possible to make a higher quality of flour; this was not used much for the common man. Although wheat has been around since the beginning, barley and rye were also used to make flour. These grains do not have as much gluten as modern wheat, but a few thousand years ago they did as well as wheat, so this bread was also commonly made. Today modern wheat has been crossbred to create thousands of varieties with higher gluten levels that it has taken over as the grain for bread. It used to be that rye or barley was the only grain that could grow well in certain environments. Now you can pick a variety of wheat that could grow almost anywhere. There is nothing wrong with barley flour or rye. They have distinct tastes which can be desirable. With the crossbreeding of these grains, they can produce somewhat more gluten than a couple of thousand years ago, but they are never going to be described as light and fluffy. Barley grain is physically hard and to remove the bran they must be pearled, which means instead of crushing the grain the bran is rubbed off.

Anyway, in the middle ages advancements in milling were made by making large stones rub together, driven by water or wind power, making flour much more plentiful and hence more bread. We had baker's yeast and wheat grain development through crossbreeding was continuing, and, although the bread may have been marginally lighter and less dense, it was still nothing like today. We had better control over the particle size, and I am going to say that most flour particle size was less than 420 microns. There was still a range of sizes, but the biggest was 420. You could just run the milled flour through the mill again and perhaps get a larger percentage of smaller grains, but this was expensive and the resulting flour more expensive, hence the common man was stuck with the first run. The first run was still better than it was 2000 years previously as to the quality of the flour, but still far from light fluffy. Now with larger mills, you can realistically separate the brain somewhat. It turns out that not only does bran make the bread darker (because of the various molecules in the bran providing its color), but also bran interfered with the rising of the bread.

As an aside, now we know why bran may interfere with the rising. For the gluten network to develop, water must be added to the proteins to get them to unfold and form a network to trap the gas. Bran fiber interferes with this protein hydration such that the gluten network is not properly activated. This may extend the time required for dough development and reduce the trapping ability of the gluten network.

Now we have centralized mills using water and air power to turn gristmills. In general, we had one pass of the grain to make the common flour. You could have flour with less bran and a more consistent and maybe smaller particle size, but you would have to pay extra. For thousands of years, people stored grain in their house and milled it as needed at home using small hand mills. As milling became a larger and more efficient industry, more people just bought flour at the market.

Most of them bought the common flour, a few rich people bought the more refined flour that could be used to make lighter bread.

Now we had a different problem as the germ in the flour (which contains much of the fat) goes bad in about six months. We figured out that if you remove the germ, the flour lasts a lot longer. So along with getting rid of the bran, millers now also got rid of the germ. I say they got rid of it, but they fed it to the livestock who liked it just fine. At this point in history, many more people are living in cities and not only stopped making their own flour, but just bought it, or just got bread from local bakeries who could use the economy of scale to sell white, light bread. If you were using a lot of flour twelve months a year, you were going to be importing flour from longer distances and needed it to have a longer shelf life. We didn't know anything about vitamins or minerals in food back then, so, it seemed like a great idea to get rid of the bran and germ to get the flour that the customers wanted.

In the mid-1800s, steam power, the steel industry and the development of the technology using roller mills to crush grain were developed. Now we had smoother wheels that could be spun faster and were more efficient in milling. Instead of crushing the seed, you could crack the husk and make the removal of the germ and bran much easier. In addition, now we could use wheat varieties that had grains that were harder (physically) and contained more gluten. We took the bran and germ left over and gave them to cattle for feed, which powered the meat industry. While we were at it, we figured out that we could use various methods to bleach the flour making it finally white, not just lighter.

Hardly anyone was grinding flour at home and now most everyone bought bread at the market. Certainly, lots of bread products such as biscuits and pastry items we made at home which required a slightly lower gluten content and a finer size particle, and dough rising was not an issue, but plenty of flour was used in the various food industries, and all of this was roller ground, degerminated, free of bran, and bleached.

In the 1920's we recognized that the germ was an important part of the nutrition and vitamins of bread. To avoid bad publicity and possible government action, the mills began adding back some of the minerals and vitamins (mainly A and B1) back to the flour. Now we have enriched flour which is said to be as good as whole wheat, but no bran, no germ which could go bad, nice and white, and good gluten content. Obviously, this is better for you than old-fashioned whole wheat.

It is not better. There are several micronutrients and minerals, as well as various molecules contained in the bran that may be necessary to maintain health and a proper gut biome. Whole wheat bread has been able to prevent starvation and provide a sustenance diet for thousands of years. I doubt if I could say the same about modern white bread. I am trying to decrease the amount of processing in my food and avoid chemicals in my diet, especially those that have not been in our diet the previous 5000 years. Later in the book I will sum up the whole purpose of the book, which is why are we getting obese and what can we do about it regarding our diet. I will discuss particle size further.

Most of the time, the germ of the grain is removed along with the bran. The germ is only about 3% of the weight of the whole grain. We already talked about fat in the germ reducing the shelf life of the flour. The germ contains essential fatty acids as well as long-chained fatty alcohols and fat-soluble vitamins (Vitamin E), along with B vitamins. The germ is the seed embryo, and hence contains all the molecular elements required to grow the plant. It also contains some sucrose and monosaccharides, but most of the energy needed to grow the plant is contained in the endosperm.

The endosperm is about 80-85% of the grain. The endosperm is surrounded by the aleurone layer, the same layer in the bran, and extends within the seed to separate the endosperm from the germ. The endosperm is primarily composed of starch granules embedded in a protein gluten matrix, but about 75% of the protein content of the grain is found in the endosperm. The endosperm is softer than bran or germ and can be milled to a very small particle size. This is useful if you are using flour with low gluten as it will give you a more even rise with smaller bubbles and less chewy texture, and you can use chemical leavening instead of yeast. This is what you want for cakes and cookies.

The endosperm contains four classes of storage protein; Globulins and albumins are a class of water-soluble proteins that have little to do with bread making. Gliadins and glutenins are insoluble in water and are the components of gluten. All of these are storage proteins, and their job is actually to provide nutrition to the growing seed. It just so happens that these gluten proteins can also facilitate the making of bread. The gluten protein gets all the press, but the albumins and globulins make the bread nutritious and contain many essential amino acids and enzymes that benefit both the digestion and nutrition of wheat. Although most of the medical problems related to bread come from the glutens, there can be a few from the globulin and albumin proteins.

Flour Treatment

We now have a fair understanding of grain. You would think that now all we have to do is somehow grind up the grain and start cooking, and in fact, that is what we did for thousands of years. Sure, there were various recipes and we put all kinds of things in bread, we even used bread for the bowls and plates. In the last few hundred years, changes have occurred in bread such that modern bread is far different from ancient bread. You may ask how that can be since it seems to be a simple process to turn grain in bread, after all, there are only four ingredients and three of them (water, salt, and yeast) seem to be pretty basic. What has changed is the flour.

We will start with the grain. We went over the traditional grains. There have probably been hundreds of thousands of varieties of wheat grains over the last six thousand years. All of them had the same basic structure, all had some measure of gluten, all could be made into some type of bread. I say all but maybe there were a few varieties that did not work out, but these probably only lasted a couple years. Farmers cross-bred crops to improve the outcome, which was usually for greater yield, resistance to pathogens, the ability to survive in different environments, and finally to make better bread. Right now, let's see how we treat the flour.

When the grain shows up at the miller, you clean it off to get rid of the bugs, dirt, and sand. We did this from the beginning. If you recall, the last thousand years we began removing bran (and germ) form the grain. This was done to produce better bread. I need to emphasize how much this desire to produce light, fluffy, white bread has affected the milling and production of the bread we eat today. All of the changes were driven by the demand of consumers to have a more edible bread, they had nothing to do with nutrition. Those of you who have tried to bake basic bread; that is buy the grain, mill it in your Vitamix or home grinder, add yeast (or sourdough starter), salt, and water; get about the same product. This is a dense, hard, dark bread that is difficult to eat. It does have a more complex flavor that modern bread, but nobody really wants to eat this type of bread. It is a basic staple that people ate for thousands of years to keep from starving.

We have tried all different ways to make this basic more palpable without using modern techniques but have had little success. One of the first ways we developed to improve the bread quality was to remove the bran and germ. (I am not counting the continual cross breeding of wheat to get more protein and thus more gluten). The millers figured out that if you tempered the grain, that is add a little water and let it rest a little while, the bran shell became harder, and the endosperm became softer. This made it easier to crack the bran into larger pieces so you could separate the bran and the germ from the endosperm easier. As the milling process became more centralized, more of this flour without bran and germ was produced making the resultant flour have a higher demand since the resultant bread was lighter and less dense. Removing the bran improves gluten development, which is the key to getting more air trapped in the dough and hence a fluffier product. This made the bread much easier to eat. This also enabled the birth of pastry products (cakes, crusts).

Pastry is flour, oil, and water with no yeast. During the 1500s these products were increasingly developed into many of the desserts we enjoy today. It was during this time centralized milling was making better (from a cooking point of view) flour. In retrospect, we recognize that it was not better from a nutritional point of view, but by now civilization had developed enough that the old type bread was not quite as essential for survival, although still important.

Tempering is still an important preparatory step before milling. Hardly anyone who grinds their own flour does this, although they could. I will review milling later, but right now I will introduce one of the oldest flour treatments, that is resting the flour. In the beginning, man probably ground up the grain into flour soon before using it. If you were doing it yourself, you did not store a bunch of flour around the house. For one thing, we figured out that whole wheat flour would go bad after a few months.

As milling became more centralized in the 1500s with waterpower turning stone wheels, part of the process required storage of the grain before milling, and storage of the flour after milling prior to its distribution. Now we know that "resting" the flour for a few weeks improves its baking quality and appearance. The flour becomes oxidized upon exposure to the air and this makes the flour a little lighter in color and improves the quality of the gluten proteins allowing more trapped air bubbles. Until modern times, this happened naturally since it took a while for the flour to end up at the final cooking destination. Now, neither mills nor bakeries store a lot of inventory, so the flour gets to the bakery within a couple of days. As we will see later, we now artificially rest the flour (this flour directly from the miller is called green flour).

There is a giant difference between what I can make at home using the four basic ingredients, and what I can buy in the store. The production of what we call modern bread (and most of us know of no other kind) from ancient bread was a slow evolution and many small steps were made over thousands of years. These steps were not taken to improve nutrition, but simply in response to customer demand in a capitalistic system. Without this demand, we would still be eating what I make at home. At this point, we still have about the same particle size of the flour grains. It won't be until the widespread implementation of roller milling that led to a much smaller average particle size, that is the main factor that I believe led to the modern obesity epidemic. Other accommodations to modern baking have added other elements that have decreased the nutritional value of bread compared to historical norms.

We have tempered the bread to make it easier to remove the bran and germ, the bakeries have gone from sourdough starter to brewer's or baker's yeast, we somewhat accidentally are resting the flour to improve gluten development and color, and the farmers are slowly developing grains with more gluten protein. By the 1800s the bread has improved texture and is softer and whiter, but still nothing like today. It is only in the last 80 years or so that modern chemistry, modern milling, and modern large-scale baking has given us modern store bread. I believe it is no coincidence that this has occurred in conjunction with modern obesity.

The goal of bakers is to sell their products. The goal of millers is to make flour bakers and the public want to buy. I'll review the additives.

Bleaching of flour is designed both to improve the appearance of flour and improves structure-forming capacity. Chemical bleaching of flour is banned in China, Europe, and Brazil. Bleaching is oxidation, which is a chemical reaction in which electrons are lost. This is usually created by the addition of oxygen atoms to a molecule. This process interrupts the chemical bonds of chromophores (various molecules that absorb certain wavelengths of light and reflect color), which creates an absence of color, and hence is seen as white. Flour normally would have a yellow color. This was initially accomplished by resting the flour and allowing atmospheric oxygen to work on the flour. This takes about a month and takes up a lot of room, so it is not surprising bakers found a chemical that could accomplish the same goal in a shorter time frame. These same oxygen molecules affect the gluten molecules in a manner which allows a better gluten formation and better rising of the dough. See chapter on gluten.

Chemical bleaching shortens this process. Basically, any white bread or white flour you buy has been chemically bleached. As we will see, the additives to flour have changed the food and added chemicals to the flour not present in the preceding 5000 years. It ends up some of these chemicals may not be good for you.

Oxidizing agents (bleaching agents)

Just like the resting of flour bleaches it somewhat and increases gluten structure, most bleaching chemicals also enhance gluten.

Benzoyl peroxide is the most common flour bleaching agent in the US. The European Union, Canada, and China have banned the use of this as a food additive because of health concerns. (liver)

Chlorine gas has also been banned in many countries. This chemical seems to enhance the formation of alloxan from the pigment molecules in the grain. Alloxan is a very potent chemical and destroys the insulin-producing cells in some animals. It has been found in about 25% of the bleached flour sold. Weakens gluten development unlike most bleaching agents, which is desirable in wafers, cakes, and cookies.

Dough Conditioners are used to either strengthen gluten formation or weaken them. They are used to make the dough more pliable and are used to enable machinery in the baking process to turn flour into bread.

Azodicarbonamide is used to make the flour appear whiter. and dough conditioner. Increases shelf life. Associated with the occurrence of the carcinogen ethyl carbamate in bread and respiratory problems. Banned in Europe, Australia

Potassium Bromide is classified as a carcinogen and is nephrotoxic in humans. Also banned in the EU and China. It is used as a dough conditioner as it strengthens gluten formation.

L Ascorbic acid is used to strengthen gluten formation. Vitamin C is destroyed by baking heat.

Acerola powder is from the acerola cherry and serves as a source of Vitamin C

Glutathione is used as a reducing agent to make doughs more manageable in baking machinery. Mainly obtained by deactivated yeasts

l-cysteine speeds up reaction withing the dough reducing bulk fermentation time. May interfere with insulin. Breaks disulfide bonds in gluten.

Calcium peroxide: dough maturing agent. Banned in China and the EU

Glycerides: crumb softening, reduce bread staling. Surfactants

Sodium stearoyl lactylate is an emulsifier which softens crumbs and allows easier mixing of ingredients. Promotes gluten.

Soya flour is milled soybeans. It is used as a conditioner in dough to make it easier to function in breadmaking machinery. It also can be used as a bleaching agent. If you have read my previous book, you know I have advised you to diminish the eating of soybean products.

Trans fats: these are hydrogenated oils of some kind that are used to improve texture and shelf life. Trans fats are artificial compounds that cannot be metabolized by your body in a normal manner. You need to avoid trans fats if at all possible, and it should be possible. Trans fats have a bad reputation, so the addition of these products is often described as "partially hydrated" something. Avoid anything that is partially hydrated.

Leavening Agent

Aluminum salts in self-rising flour leavening agent

Monocalcium phosphate (Anhydrous Monocalcium Phosphate or AMCP) Slow acting leavening agent

Sugar products are added to enhance yeast growth. These can be sucrose like molasses or cane sugar, or honey.

Preservatives

Calcium Propionate: preservative. Increases shelf life. Prevents mold growth. In mice, it stimulates glycogenolysis (sugar making) and insulin leading to weight gain in mice in human equivalent dose.

Sodium Bisulfate: preservative, enhance gluten.

Cultured wheat comes from the fermentation of wheat flour, generally with lactic acid-forming bacteria. This product provides inhibition of bacterial and mold growth. Used in place of chemicals.

Enzymes do not have to be listed in the ingredients list.

They have been used in the last 50 years to improve the rising ability of the dough. These may be able to take the place of chemicals, especially oxidizing agents, and appear to be much safer.

Malted barley dough: Malting is sprouting the grain, drying it, then grinding it for flour. Diastase is a group of enzymes that break down starches to maltose. Maltose is two glucose molecules bonded together. Maltase in the gut lining then breaks this down into glucose which is absorbed. Adding this group of enzymes increases the availability of sugar for the yeast, hence promoting rising.

Amylase is an enzyme produced by yeast and added to flour to enable the conversion of starch to maltose. Alpha-amylase only acts on damaged and gelatinized starch. Alpha-amylase breaks the chain of glucose molecules into smaller pieces, while beta-amylase breaks maltose units (two molecules of glucose) off at the end of the chain. Found in wheat grains. Activated when exposed to water. Most of the action occurs at broken or smaller sized starch granules which have a higher surface area. The yeast also contains maltase and can absorb a maltose molecule and break in down into glucose units. Yeast contain amylases but it takes time to produce enough of these enzymes to break down significant quantities of starch. Amylase may not appear on the ingredient list.

Protease breaks peptide bonds between amino acids in a protein and exists in flour, yeast, and malt. Too much of it breaks down gluten. A little softens dough and makes it workable. It provides amino acids for yeast to process and form into flavor compounds. These enzymes are also produced by the lactic acid bacteria in sourdough. The breakdown of proteins in higher in sourdough. The bacteria in sourdough have the capacity to breakdown the toxic proteins involved in celiac disease.

Transglutaminase is a naturally occurring enzyme that encourages the cross-linking reaction between gluten and other protein molecules; as such it improves the gluten properties of bread. It performs a function similar to the way oxidizing chemical improve gluten in dough, but without the chemicals.

Vital Wheat Gluten: This is a product made from wheat dough in which everything else is removed but the gluten protein. This protein is used as a meat replacement in Seitan. It is often added to low protein flours such as rye to provide extra rising. When I go to the store and look at the organic 100% whole wheat flour that is much less dense than the bread I make at home, there is always additional wheat gluten added in addition to extra sugar and enzymes.

Nobody even heard of these agents 200 years ago. They have been incorporated into almost all processed bread to enable faster baking, better rising, better texture, and to enable the machinery involved in baking to function economically. They also were created to shorten the time required to rest flour, shorten the time for bread to rise, and shorten the time to mix the flour and knead the dough. None of these enhance the nutrition of the bread.

It appears that for thousands of years we have been trying to develop means of producing lighter, less dense, easier to eat, easier to eat, cheaper to make, and more economical ways to produce flour and bread. In doing so, we have gone far beyond the four basic ingredients needed to make bread. For thousands of years, there was very slow progress in the milling of bread. With the industrial age, milling made rapid advances including the creation of roller milling; all with the goal of producing this fluffy, white bread.

Modern bread is a different food from historical bread; both in nutrition, content, and taste.

Since almost everyone buys flour, let's go over what you see in the store:

Start with whole wheat. You now know that this can be made from roller mills or stone mills. In the roller mills, the bran and germ are removed, the endosperm milled, and everything put back together at the end. These particles are of consistent size and smaller than stone-milled flour. You can make bread that is slightly dark, lighter than the 2000-year-old bread, and slightly denser than fluffy bread. Look at the adjectives for other properties.

You can also find stone-ground flour. This may be described as 100% whole wheat. Often it is organic. It is usually sifted such that no particles are larger than 420 microns. (about half a millimeter)

All-purpose flour is the most widely used flour. This is a mixture of high-gluten hard wheat flour and low-gluten soft wheat flour. The percentage of protein can be adjusted but it is usually between 9% and 11%. It may be enriched and bleached. It is white.

Bread flour: This does come in white or whole wheat varieties. The protein content is 11%-13%. As the name implies, this is used to make bread and we want a little more gluten.

Cake and pastry flour: These have a lower protein content, 8%-9%. You don't want a chewy pastry, but rather fluffy and tender. Often chlorinated.

Self-rising flour: This often has lower protein. Added baking soda and baking soda allows a slight rise of the dough without a lot of gluten. Typically used for biscuits.

Semolina: This is a high protein, coarse (average particle size for medium coarse is 375 microns) flour made with durum wheat and often used in the making of pasta. It is made from Durum wheat. There is a finer version of semolina called durum flour which is not often used for bread. This flour has not changed much in a thousand years except for additives.

Now the adjectives associated with your flour buys:

Bleached flour means a whitening agent has been added, and probably the germ and bran removed. Some bleaching agents affect gluten development If chlorine gas is used, the adjective "chlorinated" may be used.

Enriched means some nutrients are returned to the flour after milling.

Hard flour means a higher protein content.

Gluten flour is just refined gluten protein (100% protein). Since whole wheat flour contains bran which may inhibit gluten formation, gluten flour may be added to get better rising.

Assume flour is non-organic if not labeled organic. Unfortunately, the meaning of organic can be a moving target, so you may need to read the teeny fine print.

Sprouted grain flour: this is made by allowing the grain to sprout (grow for a couple of days), dry the grain, then make it into flour. This process releases amino acids, vitamins, and micronutrients. It also begins breaking down the starch molecules (which are long chains of glucose molecules) into maltose (which are two glucose molecules bonded together).

After all, the sprouting process is getting nutrients to the newly grown plants and these nutrients need to be readily available. Sprouting does increase the vitamins, essential amino acids, and modifies the gluten proteins which may help some gluten-sensitive people. It also decreases the phytic acid, which can bind to the minerals and prevent absorption. You can buy sprouted flour or bread made with sprouted flour. Of course, this is going to be whole wheat, since you must start with a seed. Most will be stone milled.

Yeast

There are three other ingredients other than flour in risen bread. I will go over these briefly.

This book is *Bread for the Modern Diet*. Bread has a larger definition than simply a loaf of wheat. Although I have confined the discussion to wheat gluten products, it is important to remember that all kinds of products are made of wheat grain other than risen bread. Of course, flatbreads have been known since the beginning. These can be made with all kinds of non-wheat; non-gluten flours and we eat them often in the form of corn flatbreads or tacos. These do not require yeast. Batters, which constitute the category of biscuits, cookies, cake, and pastry, also do not require yeast. The underlying theme of this book and the previous one is: what has occurred in our diet the last hundred years that has led to obesity and its metabolic consequences? Insulin resistance seems to be a major factor, and carbohydrate ingestion drives insulin resistance.

I have attempted to answer how our carbohydrate ingestion has changed, how our carbohydrates have changed, and how our processing of food has changed to lead us to our current dietary epidemic. Bread (or at least grain consumption), has always been a major component of the human diet. The basis of bread is flour. This chapter is about yeast, which is a component of risen bread, but the same flour is used for non-risen bread and other flour products such as cakes and cookies. So, despite having no yeast, they still have flour.

Yeast is a single-cell organism that is a part of the fungus family. They can preserve themselves in a spore form and are present throughout our environment. In fact, to use yeast as the leavening agent in sourdough, one only has to leave wet dough exposed to air for a day, and you get a yeast colony-forming. A leavening agent is a substance that causes the expansion of dough by the release of gases in the mixture. When man first ground wheat and added water, he noticed that if you left this around for a while, the dough started rising. Cook a patty of this on a hot rock, and it tasted much better than just soggy flour.

Now let's review photosynthesis. A plant can take carbon dioxide (CO_2) and water (H_2O), add sunlight (energy), and make sugar ($C_6H_{12}O_6$) and oxygen (O_2). The plant can then take this sugar molecule and attach it to a bunch of other sugar molecules to make starch. It can then store this starch so that when it needs energy to make something else, it can perform the reverse of this reaction and get energy, water, and carbon dioxide. We can cheat and get this energy for the plants by stealing the starch they already made from sunlight and converting it back into energy and carbon dioxide. This is basically how every living thing gets energy (except a few odd bacteria). Now some of the time we start with more complex substances and do not break them down completely, but energy from the sun is the basis for animal energy.

Fermentation is a metabolic process that produces chemical changes in organic substances for the extraction of energy. In yeast the metabolic processes are set up such that to extract energy for life, the yeast cell can take a sugar molecule and convert it into two ethanol (alcohol) molecules and two carbon dioxide molecules. This gas is trapped in the gluten complex and you get risen dough. In real life, this is what mainly happens, but a hundred other different types of chemicals are also produced. For our purposes, carbon dioxide is the main product. The alcohol is easily evaporated in breadmaking and does not contribute to the flavor.

A simpler form of fermentation can be performed by some bacteria in which they take a glucose molecule and turn it into two lactate molecules (but no gas) and energy. This will be important in sourdough bread. I am making this simple, but life is very complex. A few other different molecules are always being made either by using an alternate means of breaking down the sugar molecule or recombining some of the products differently. There are many different bacteria, they all need energy, and they get it by breaking down molecules in different ways resulting in many different products. If you break down sugar to its simplest elements, you end up where we started with carbon dioxide and water.

There are three main categories of yeast that we can practically consider. These are Natural yeast, baker's yeast, and brewer's yeast. We start with natural yeast which is used in the making of sourdough bread. Yeast seems to be around almost everywhere, and natural yeast is found in the air, on the grain, even on the hands of the people making bread. This natural yeast leavening was by far the most common yeast used for making risen bread. It was usually used as a starter solution, in which a small amount of a solution containing yeast (and bacteria) was maintained by adding flour and water to a fermented mixture. This allowed one to always have yeast on hand, and you could maintain this starter mixture by just adding flour and water every few days. This gave you a head start in making bread in that instead of having to wait around a day or two for a natural culture to reach the point where there was enough yeast present to use it effectively, you could start cooking in a few hours. Natural yeast adds different flavors to the bread depending on the species, and since there are lots of different kinds of yeast that can be found in the environment, there can be many different flavors, often quite subtle.

The difference between sourdough bread and store-bought bread is the presence of lactic acid-forming bacteria in the starter. Like yeast, bacteria are all around us. The starter is a solution of yeast and bacteria that can form lactic acid. The yeast causes the dough to rise, and the bacterial lactic acid causes the sourness in the dough. The bacteria can metabolize some of the sugars the yeast cannot, and the yeast can ferment the byproduct of the bacteria which is lactic acid. Both benefit as bacteria get energy from leftover sugars, and the yeast can metabolize the lactic acid, hence preventing its buildup which would eventually slow down the bacterial growth.

Of course, this whole process is much more complicated. Remember that the whole grain contains a lot of different kinds of sugar in the germ and bran; some of these cannot be used by the yeast. During the fermentation with yeast, many different chemicals are formed either as intermediaries or as a result of biochemical processes. These can affect the final taste. Many of these may also be fermented by the bacteria, again resulting in different molecules being formed. The bacteria may also be able to break down the proteins in the grain, both resulting in amino acids, and forming intermediate proteins. The specific species of yeast or bacteria can be different in different starters, and they can also change depending on the environment.

Your starter may be completely different from your neighbor, but they have in common yeast and a bacterium that forms lactic acid. If you recall, I mentioned phytates are present in the bran and germ. Phytates can bind minerals and prevent their absorption in the gut. Lactic acid can prohibit the formation of this complex and increase the availability of the minerals present. Basically, the bread is pre-digested. This may delay the rapid absorption of glucose, such that sourdough bread does have a lower glycemic index than other types of bread, meaning a slower rise in the glucose level. Now we a looking at organic, stone-ground, whole wheat, sourdough bread as appearing to be the healthiest in our diet, and probably the most commonly eaten bread the last 5000 years.

The next yeast on the list is brewer's yeast. We have been drinking alcohol since soon after creation. Man has made alcohol out of almost every plant that contains enough sugar. We are looking for yeast that will convert sugar into ethanol. We don't mind if there is a little carbonation. Ethanol is a result of fermentation, which is a method by which animals obtain energy by converting the sugar into smaller molecules with the ensuing release of energy. Yeast is great at this.

Bread, beer, and wine probably all came about around the same time. Although you can use almost any yeast to make alcohol, some do a much better job than others. Since alcohol is a byproduct of yeast fermentation, eventually too high a level will kill the yeast. The fermentation process for making alcohol takes much longer than the few hours to get bread to rise, and many other chemicals have the chance to be formed. The various alcoholic beverages depend upon the source of the sugar used: Beer uses grain, wine uses grapes, fruits are used to make all kinds on brandy, mead uses honey, rum uses sugarcane.

To enhance the production of sugar molecules (remember starch is a long chain of glucose and amylase is the enzyme that breaks down starch), the grain in beer is often germinated to increase the amount of amylase present (malted). The making of beer requires yeast, and it did not take long for brewers to figure out how to maintain a supply of yeast, after all, there was a lot left over after the beer was made. If you lived near a brewery, it was easy to get yeast to make bread and thus you did not have to keep your own sour bread starter around. This fresh yeast spoiled after a couple of days and you must have a continuing supply. The brewers were always trying to get yeast that would make more alcohol or impart a better flavor, while the bakers were trying to get yeast that would make a fast rise and may impart a different flavor. That led us to baker's yeast. Believe it or not, some people did not like the taste of sourdough bread from natural yeast.

Yeast contains amylase which enables the digestion of the starch in the grain into maltose (two glucose molecules) Yeast also contains maltase, which allows the splitting of maltose into glucose. It takes a while to get enough amylase so that bakers figured out, they could just add sugar of some kind to get the process going faster. They could also add some malted grain. Malted grain is grain to which water has been added to stimulate the growth of the seed. One of the first processes to occur is to get amylase activated as the seed needs energy first. Hence allowing the grain to sprout a little, drying out and grinding the grain, and adding it to the flour gives you a boost of amylase.

The bakers and the brewers had a close relationship and were always developing different yeasts. They were both relying on the fermentation process. About 100 years ago, Fleischmann's Yeast company began operating and changed the ball game. They developed granulated dry yeast that did not require refrigeration and thus had a long shelf life. Now the bakers were independent of the brewers and the company began developing yeast specifically for bread making. Today we go down to the store and but some packets of yeast. If you bake a lot of bread, you can buy it in bulk. If you are a bakery, you may be able to use fresh yeast. The yeast you buy causes bread to rise much faster than the sourdough starter.

To complete the subject, I will mention baking soda and baking powder. Baking soda is sodium bicarbonate and produces carbon dioxide gas when an acid material is added. This is the same carbon dioxide gas produced by yeast. It is released more rapidly than the gas produced by yeast and used with thin batters which are cooked quickly (pancakes). Usually, an acidic ingredient in the batter activates the baking soda. It can also be released when exposed to temperatures above 176 degrees. Baking soda is sodium bicarbonate (baking soda) with another acidifying agent added to it so that no acidic ingredient is required. Both baking powder and baking soda provide carbon dioxide to raise whatever dough or batter you are using. Both release this gas more rapidly than yeast so that after mixing, cooking should not be delayed.

SALT

Salt is one of the basic ingredients in bread. It adds taste by possibly affecting your taste buds, but no matter how it works, it enhances the flavor of food. Also, the sodium and chloride atoms assist in the formation of gluten which enhances the rise of the dough, a goal we seem to have been working toward since the beginning. By holding onto water, it can prevent the bread from going stale as quickly. Of course, in a humid environment, your bread can become soggy. It appears that all normal sale (NaCl) works as long as the particles are small enough to dissolve.

Not only is salt required for taste, but the negatively charged chloride atoms can also bond with the positively charged gluten structure to neutralize some of the charges and allow the positive charge gluten filaments to bind more closely together. Now, how much salt do you need to add? We have many articles telling us to cut down on salt for various reasons. It ends up that eating a lot of bread can contribute to your general salt intake. The advice often is based upon the weight of the baked product. I am going to advise you to weigh the amount of flour you use and use 2% of that weight for the amount of salt you put in. That's still too complicated so this is an example using a combination of good old American units and metric units this is what we have.

1 cup of flour is about 120 grams.

2% of 120 grams is 2.4 grams.

One teaspoon of salt weighs 6 grams

So, if you used four cups of flour to make a small loaf of bread, you would add 9.6 grams of salt.

This is about 1 ½ teaspoon of salt.

Unlike many measurements in baking, this amount does not have to be exact, but at least close.

WATER

The process of making bread is an extremely complicated chemical reaction that is even now not well understood. You have a chemical soup with water being the basis for that soup. The enzymes in the wheat grains are dormant, as are the starch granules, until exposure to water. There are numerous enzymes and micronutrients required to begin the process of germination. When water is applied to the grain, the seeds begin to initiate germination, and if you are malting the grain, your wait for a small sprout to form. With the addition of yeast and lactic acid bacteria in sourdough, we begin many biological processes, all requiring an aqueous solution and producing a wide variety of biochemicals, many requiring minerals. The process is complicated by the changing pH of the solution (dough), the varying availability of oxygen, the changing temperature, the changing availability of water molecules as some get absorbed or used up in chemical reactions, and finally the physical deformation of the solution which changes its biochemical composition (kneading). The information I have provided you is a great simplification as to the actual chemical processes occurring. It would require many crowded blackboards to chemically depict what is really happening.

Water starts the ball rolling. It is better not to use chlorinated water as we want the yeast and bacteria to grow. After milling, the bran and germ are in smaller pieces such that water molecules can bind to molecules and activate the enzymatic processes as well as dissolve the various chemicals and proteins present to allow interactions. The endosperm is composed of protein and starch, and this deserves a more detailed look. The large starch molecules come in two forms, one linear called amylose, one highly branched called amylopectin. Alpha and Beta amylose then digest these large molecules into the two carbon maltose molecules which are then split into individual glucose molecules. When water is added to starch, it is absorbed in the spaces between starch particles which leads to swelling.

If you added enough water and heated the solution, you would burst the starch particles and form a gravy. We are not using that much water in our bread baking. In our usage, water enters the tightly bound regions in the amylopectin which are in a crystallized structure. As heat is applied, the amylose chains begin to separate, and the starch structure becomes more disorganized such that water can penetrate and dissolve the granules. The temperature at which the starch gelatinized varies based upon the plant type of starch, the amount of water present, the pH, the concentration of salt, sugar, fat, and protein in the recipe, and the particle size(broken granules) which depends on the milling process. When we make bread, these are dynamic conditions. We can add chemicals that can dramatically change the process.

During cooling, this gelatinized starch can reform amylose bonds and harden or set. The condition of the starch varies with temperature. As the temperature rises, changes in the starch structures result in varying degrees of viscosity. Viscosity is a quality of a semifluid condition which describes the internal friction of the matter. In other words, if the matter can move around easily, it has less internal friction. If you have to force it around (say like kneading dough), it has greater internal friction and hence more viscosity. The harder it is to stir the mixture, the more viscosity. In bread this condition is changing all the time depending on how much water is present, which dissolves the starch, the temperature, which unravels the starch granules, and the presents of other ingredients in the solution. We kind of want the dough to have a lower viscosity as gas is produced by the yeast to get a good rise, and we want it to eventually set to prevent all this good rise from going flat.

A lot of this process is related to the gelatinization of starch and the retrogradation of starch, which is the starch going in the other direction and becoming less viscous. We need the starch to be released, we need the starch to be digested to provide sugar to the yeast, we need the starch to be elastic enough to encompass the gas bubbles, and we need the starch to eventually set to keep the structure of the bread

from collapsing. At the same time, too much water will weaken the ability of the bread to rise.

At the same time, we have gluten development which allows the dough to stretch which allows the dough to trap the gas and provides some chewiness and crumb structure. Gluten has its own chemical processes going on that interact with starch gelatinization and retrogradation. We started out with four simple ingredients that mankind figured out from the beginning could be combined to form a nutritious food, one that could enable you to survive during times of food shortage with that food alone, which the ingredients could be stored for years.

Through trial and error, we developed various formulations of bread, both for variety and in an attempt to make it more palatable. It appeared we liked it better when it was less dense and easier to eat, and slowly over thousands of years we progressed toward this goal. In the process, we made bread, the historical last resort to prevent starvation, less nutritious, highly processed, and adulterated with chemicals to the point that now it is as white, fluffy, sweet, long-lasting, and versatile as we want; But can we now live on bread and water? Instead of preventing starvation, is flour now a factor in obesity and diabetes?

GLUTEN

By now everyone has heard of gluten. More specifically, everyone has heard of gluten-free. This means that whatever gluten is, this product does not have any. Before we start talking about gluten-free, let's see what gluten is.

As we spoke about earlier, the properties of gluten allow us to have bread that is not as dense and has a more palatable grain texture. It turns out that wheat contains a lot of gluten, which is simply a group of proteins that have an elastic property so that it may contain any carbon dioxide produced by the yeast and hence cause the dough to rise upon warming of the yeast. The more rising, the less dense the product.

You can make flour out of all kinds of grains and legumes, but only wheat, rye, and barley contain enough gluten to enable the bread to rise. I will talk about oats later. Leavened bread usually means that yeast is present. You can also have chemical leavening (baking powder) that can cause a slight rise. You can have all the yeast you want, but if you don't have gluten, you get flatbread.

Nowadays we can buy gluten-free risen bread, but that means we don't use grains with gluten, and that we add something else like xanthan gum (a product of the bacteria *Xanthomonas campestris* grown in a sugar solution) or guar gum (made from the guar bean plant). These replicate the elastic properties of gluten but give the bread a slightly different taste.

Almost all the bread eaten in the United States is from wheat and thus contains gluten. I am going to go into a little biochemistry in which the nomenclature is quite confusing. It is almost like this was done intentionally. Anyone with common sense can follow the steps, it's just that now we learn a little foreign language. This seems to be true of almost all sciences. It sounds hard because we just don't know the language. Anyway, my job is to teach you.

Gluten is composed of two different types of proteins:

PROLAMINS

(Plant storage proteins having a high proline amino acid content)

AND

GLUTELINS

(these also form the network that hold starch granules in the
endosperm)

The prolamins are different in wheat, rye, barley, and oats.

WHEAT = GLIADINS

BARLEY = HORDEINS

RYE = SECALIN

OATS = AVENIN

These are groups of proteins. Remember I told you that wheat dough is composed of wheat grain with three sets of chromosomes. Each set may code for slightly different proteins, so that with each variety of wheat grain the composition of proteins may be slightly different. I will just talk about wheat gluten. That means this group of Prolamins proteins in wheat is called Gliadins. Let me replace Prolamins with Gliadins since I am only talking about wheat. Now we have:

GLUTEN is composed of:

GLIADINS

(the group of prolamins in wheat. If this were barley or rye, it would
be hordeins or secalin)

AND

GLUTELINS

Pay attention to the ends of these words as they are all going to sound alike. I wonder if this was done intentionally to make it harder to understand. Sometimes they call the whole group of prolamin proteins gluten proteins, regardless of which grain the prolamin came from.

Just like the Prolamin proteins in wheat are called GLIADINS, the Glutelin proteins in wheat are called GLUTENINS. Barley and Rye glutelins are just called barley glutelin and rye glutelin. Now we have:

GLUTEN in wheat is composed of:
GLIADINS
AND
GLUTENINS

If this were barely or rye, this would be barley glutelin rye glutelin)

Gluten is formed when the glutenin protein molecules cross-link to form a network attached to gliadin molecules. This increases the elasticity and thickness of the dough, allowing the yeast's carbon dioxide to be trapped in the dough and make it less dense. Throughout history and to this day, people like their beards to be lighter and less dense. Most of the bread that is sold is not dense and heavy but rather light and airy.

Most of the problems that drive the creation of gluten-free bread lie in the gliadin component of gluten. The gliadins can be separated into four groups: alpha, beta, gamma, and omega gliadins. These, in turn, are associated with different types of anti-inflammatory diseases, including celiac disease. I will talk about why gluten-free bread exists in the next chapter. Rye, Barley, and Oats may all be said to contain gluten, but this is not the wheat gluten we are talking about since the prolamin proteins are different. Nevertheless, we call it gluten and speak of them just as we would wheat gluten.

Now is the time to talk about oats. Technically oats contain gluten, but this is not the same as gluten in wheat, barley, or rye. It does not produce a gluten network that enables bread to rise, hence oat bread always has a better gluten source added. When we say gluten-free oat flour, what we mean is that this flour does not contain any contaminants (or very little) of gluten from wheat, barley or rye. Oats are hulled and this must be removed before eating. The de-hulled grain is called oat groats. This is the whole grain. You can soak this in water, cook them, and eat them as they are. Needless to say, these have a large particle size. You can steam the groats and press them between rollers to get rolled oats. The advantage is that they can cook faster and have a different texture. You can also get steel-cut oats in which you just chop the groats into little pieces. These have a little longer cooking time than rolled and a different texture. Instant oats are the most processed and are pre-cooked, dried, rolled, and pressed thinner than rolled oats. These cook faster and are soft and mushy.

Oats are a grain and are just as good for you as wheat bread. Their disadvantage is that they are not as portable. You could cook up a loaf of bread four thousand years ago, put it in a sack, and use that for food the next few days if you were traveling. A bag of oats was not quite as portable and you would have to cook them as needed, although you could just chew the groats. Like hulled wheat, the hulled oats could be stored for a long time and used to prevent starvation. Oats like cool, wet summers so were popular in Ireland and the Scandinavian cultures. Since historical records are from the middle east and oats did not grow as well there, they did not catch on so that there is not as much historical information as wheat. Regardless, the usage of bread is just too handy.

Oats are not really gluten-free. It has some gluten, although with some different proteins than wheat and some with gluten sensitivity can tolerate them without reactions. This is always going to be a trial by fire approach. If you have real, severe celiac disease, don't try it. If you think you have a little gluten sensitivity, you may be able to tolerate oats and they are a great addition to a nutritious diet. At the end I will wrap up how we have corrupted wheat bread from its beginnings and how processing of flour has contributed to our obesity epidemic, I can't say the same thing about oats. The processing does not lead to small particle size and the use of oat flour is minuscule compared to wheat flour. There are almost no chemical additives. Unfortunately, they are rather bland and do not provide the flavor of wheat bread. Oats are underutilized in the modern diet. Oats are rich in soluble fiber which I will discuss toward the end.

Back to gluten. Wheat, Rye, and Barley are the only plants that contain gluten such that bread can be made of the flour that can contain air, and hence be classified as risen bread. The gluten enables the dough to trap gas that can give the final product a crumb structure that is not dense, as well as contribute to the overall formation of taste. The ability to grain to be stored for long periods has prevented starvation throughout history. The ability of gluten has enabled flour to be fermented by yeast and cooked, making the protein and carbohydrate readily available and digestible. All due to gluten.

Gluten is not a single protein but a group of proteins. There are many varieties of bread which means there are many different genes in bread. This means that the proteins making up gluten may not all be identical in different varieties. Therefore, when I say gluten, it is not a singular protein but rather a family of proteins that all together can create a protein network that is both elastic and plastic, and therefore permit the bread to rise. Rye and barley do not form as strong a gluten network as wheat.

Gluten is described as both elastic; meaning if stretched it will try to return to its original shape, and plastic; meaning it will deform under pressure without tearing. The dough can now expand under the pressure of the carbon dioxide produced by the yeast yet stretch so that the gas cannot escape. If the dough were just elastic, the gas would just accumulate in a few large pockets. Just plastic and gas would escape the dough. There needs to be a balance of these properties to give us light, fluffy bread.

The water-soluble albumin and globulin proteins account for about 20% of the protein in flour, the insoluble gluten proteins (gliadins and glutenins) account for the rest. The gluten proteins are quite large, from a few thousand amino acids up to a million. If you add in a few million water molecules, the interaction becomes quite complicated and is not completely understood. These proteins are long-chained, sometimes coiled, may have different side chains, may be folded back on itself or intertwined with itself or other proteins, and can be chemically bonded to itself or other proteins. Gluten proteins do not dissolve in water, but water molecules can fill spaces between the tangle of proteins.

When water is mixed with flour, the proteins begin to untangle as the water molecules separate the gluten molecules by forming hydrogen bonds. The kneading of bread, which is necessary to form an organized gluten network, aligns these molecules as they are unfolded, and thus facilitates cross-linking between the protein chains, which stiffens the dough. There is still some coiling of the molecules, and this contributes to the elasticity of the dough. As you straighten the molecules through kneading, the coiled topography tends to pull them back together. Fat in the flour and salt molecules affect the cross-linking in multiple ways that can either strengthen the cross-linking bonds or weaken them. The bonds between gluten molecules often involve sulfur atoms and these bonds can be broken or even encouraged with the physical manipulation of the environment (kneading). It is even possible to break down the gluten network by over kneading (although this is unlikely if you aren't using machinery).

Gluten Sensitivity

It has become apparent that certain conditions and symptoms may be relieved by eliminating gluten in the diet. For the most part, these conditions involve some type of activation of the immune system which can inflict both direct damages to the villi lining the gut as well as causing various systemic effects. There also appears to be a category of symptomatic disorders whereby gut symptoms appear to resolve with the elimination of gluten in the diet, despite not being able to prove an immune system connection.

Serious diseases such as celiac disease, gluten ataxia, and dermatitis herpetiformis may require several diagnostic tests (including a biopsy) to determine the correct diagnosis. These are autoimmune diseases and are nothing to screw around with. It is important to treat them vigorously. Fortunately, these are a small percentage of those presenting with possible gluten sensitivity.

There is also a classification of gluten sensitivity known as wheat allergy. This can be considered more like a food allergy, or hay fever. There are many proteins in wheat to which allergies can develop. Like other allergies, sometimes it is difficult to track down the specific protein. This is an immunoglobin E related immune response, unlike celiac disease.

Finally, we have Non-celiac gluten (wheat) sensitivity which is a separate category, and a spectrum of symptoms that seem to be relieved by a reduction of gluten in the diet. A diagnosis of celiac disease and wheat allergy must be eliminated to get this diagnosis. A common denominator of all these conditions is that the removal of gluten in the diet improves the symptoms. Let's look at each of these categories.

Celiac Disease

This is a chronic autoimmune disease that causes intestinal villi destruction. The manifestations of this disease revolve around the malabsorption of nutrients caused by this destruction. Historically this was identified in children in whom the failure to thrive and gain weight more easily manifested. The consequences of this malabsorption also included diarrhea, abdominal distention/discomfort, and abnormal stool; these symptoms resulting from the bacterial fermentation and digestion of the unabsorbed nutrients. This also leads to deficiencies in various vitamins and minerals with resulting health consequences. The symptoms are subtle and often results in several years before the correct diagnosis is made. In adults, this may only be manifested by fatigue or anemia, with no or vague intestinal complaints, and often may be confused with irritable bowel syndrome. To review:

Wheat Gluten = Gliadins and Glutenins

The Gliadins can be further broken down into:

a(alpha) and b(beta) gliadins

Y(gamma) gliadins

w(omega) gliadins

These are elements to which the immune system reacts and results in the subsequent destruction of villi and malabsorption. As a result of the chronic inflammation-induced, other immunologic diseases become more manifest. One of the results of this inflammation is that larger proteins may be absorbed instead of digested into amino acids. These proteins may further activate the immune system against proteins that may be similar to your normal tissue, and result in various immune complexes diseases.

Celiac disease was recognized for hundreds of years and often called sprue, a malnutrition syndrome. The connection with gluten was not well recognized till studies after the Dutch Famine 1944-1945 showed that children hospitalized for malabsorption syndrome improved as wheat was not available. In the ensuing years, gluten was identified as the cause and a gluten-free diet was found to be the only effective treatment for this condition.

Celiac disease is a genetic disease. A gene is inherited which makes receptors on immune cells that determine if a substance is foreign to the body more sensitive to the gluten proteins. This revs up the immune system to begin an immune response to the villi in the intestines. Stopping exposure to these proteins diminishes the immune response over time. Most celiac patients improve markedly after stopping the ingestion of gluten. Like everything else in the human body, people are slightly different, and some require absolutely no gluten to get better, others just a marked decrease in intake.

The diagnosis is not particularly easy. There is a test that, if it is negative, means you probably don't have the disease. We can test for anti-transglutaminase antibodies which is positive in the majority of celiac patients. The disease has a spectrum of severity which makes it difficult to absolutely make the diagnosis based on one test. Even a biopsy of intestinal villi can be ambiguous. The importance of making the diagnosis is that the treatment must be adhered to throughout one's life. Celiac does not get better on its own and gluten avoidance must be vigorously enforced.

Dermatitis herpetiformis

This is also a chronic autoimmune disease characterized by a blistering skin condition that can be intensely itchy. It is a cutaneous manifestation of celiac disease, involving the same type genes. Anti-transglutaminase antibodies now affect the skin instead of the villi. Various medications can provide some symptomatic improvement, but like celiac, a gluten-free diet is the mainstay of treatment. These individuals have concomitant villi injury. Biopsy material is much easier to obtain and those with this manifestation of the disease have an easier time getting a firm diagnosis of celiac. About one percent of people may have some degree of celiac, less than 0.1% have skin manifestations.

Gluten ataxia

I include this condition because it is also treated with a gluten-free diet, and it is presumed to also be an autoimmune disease triggered by the ingestion of gluten. Ataxia is a condition with gait abnormality, incoordination, or tremor and is a result of the death of neurons in the cerebellum. It is not a celiac disease and celiac disease does not progress to ataxia. Less than 10% of people with this condition present with any gastrointestinal symptoms, although about 40% can be shown to have some intestinal damage. This appears to arise from a different variant of the genes that produce susceptibility to celiac disease, yet the treatment is the same. I include this rare disease because if the neurons die, they don't grow back, and extreme gluten avoidance needs to start right now.

Wheat Allergy

This is the second of the three groups of diseases that we treat with the gluten-free diet; although, wheat allergy does not have to involve the gluten proteins, but rather one of the many other proteins in wheat. Remember there are water-soluble globulin and albumin proteins in wheat as well as gluten proteins. In some with wheat allergy, you may have to avoid all wheat products, not just gluten. Small amounts of rye or barley may not cause any problems. Wheat allergy is not celiac.

Symptoms of wheat allergy are similar to other food allergies and include eczema, hives, asthma, allergic rhinitis abdominal cramping, nausea, and vomiting. Unlike celiac, these symptoms arise soon after exposure to wheat or gluten (which is just one of the groups of proteins in wheat). Asthma may also be related to wheat allergy, along with wheat dust and pollen.

Wheat allergy may be quite complicated to track down. There are about 30,000 to 50,000 different wheat varieties and there are many subtle differences between the proteins made (as each to these varieties have a different genome). Most wheat in the US comes from about 500 to 1000 different varieties. You may be buying hard red winter wheat, but two adjacent fields may have a different variety. You may be allergic to the wheat in one field, but not the next. Often these proteins may be slightly different (maybe one amino acid) but will cross-react with the immune system. Although the gluten from different varieties may be different, they are close enough that avoiding gluten, in general, may be enough.

I will mention the rare condition of exercise-induced anaphylaxis. Anaphylaxis is a life-threatening allergic response (Use the EpiPen). It is not well understood but exercise has something to do with it. A subset of this condition is when exercise only invokes this reaction when the ingestion of a food allergen previously took place. Wheat is one of the common trigger foods, and the element responsible may be that omega gliadin in wheat gluten I showed you earlier. Celiacs are sensitive to alpha, beta, and gamma gliadins.

Non-Celiac Gluten (or Wheat) Sensitivity

This is a somewhat nebulous clinical entity in which the ingestion of gluten leads to intestinal and/or extraintestinal symptoms that improve once gluten-containing foods have been removed from the diet. For this diagnosis to be made, celiac disease and wheat allergy must have been excluded from the diagnosis.

There is no biological marker for this condition and the diagnosis is based upon the improvement of the symptoms once the treatment (decreasing gluten in the diet) has been initiated. As you can imagine, there may be a placebo component in this treatment.

There are many people with digestive or intestinal disorders. They have bloating or cramping after eating. They may have fatigue that cannot be explained. It may be that headaches, constipation, diarrhea, depression, emotional lability may be present without any other particular diagnosis. I would not be surprised if diet were a contributing factor to many of these difficult to diagnose conditions. Our diet today is markedly different from history and there is no doubt that the incidence of obesity, diabetes, autoimmune disease, and cancer is increasing. Our diet now contains high fructose corn syrup, processed sugar, soybean, various chemicals and preservatives, and very different processing methods than were used the majority of human history.

Gluten sensitivity can be indistinguishable from irritable bowel syndrome, a condition that includes abdominal pain and changes in bowel movement patterns. There is an association between anxiety, depression, and fatigue. There is much communication between the brain and gut, and disorders on either may affect the other.

I cannot ignore these symptoms as it appears almost half of the patients have some element of these symptoms. It does no good to say it is psychological because, even if it is, what do you do about it? You must address the reasons that drive the patient to see you.

First, we must address celiac disease. This is a serious condition and no matter what other symptoms you have, we must stop gluten ingestion. Failure to do this will lead to serious health problems. Second, let us eliminate food allergies. Often this will occur soon after eating the offending food and the connection can be made. Finally examine the patient to try to eliminate a diagnosable condition associated with a treatment, or a psychological condition that may require medication. We then may still be left with a large number of people who "just don't feel right" and whose current condition is affecting their life adversely.

Diet therapy is a logical starting point to treat this condition. Treating obesity and prediabetes may go a long way toward improving health. I have already written a book, *Diabetes, Prediabetes, Obesity: Diagnosis, prevention, and treatment*. Addressing this issue may improve the quality of life in these patients.

Even if we treat obesity/prediabetes, patients may still experience some of these GI symptoms. Food elimination diets may be attempted and can sometimes be a fruitful approach. In modern times, elimination of gluten from the diet has become a practical treatment that a patient can adopt with little oversight. In man's history, this may have been more difficult, and in fact, could have threatened survival since grain has traditionally been the food category stored for lean times, and stopping wheat intake may have led to malnutrition. Now, that is not the case, and eliminating gluten is not a detriment to a healthy diet.

I have added an addendum discussing wheat germ agglutinin (WGA). It is likely that a few of the gluten sensitive patients may actually be sensitive to wheat germ agglutinin, and thus may be able to eat gluten without a problem but not whole wheat bread which contains the WGA. Since white flour is bleached and the bran and germ removed, there is little WGA left, and these patients may be able to eat this type bread without difficulty.

MODERN DIET

We all probably have sucrose in our diet, but the main source of glucose in the diet of humans (and most other animals) is starch. Starch is a long chain of glucose molecules and is the way plants store energy, and what we eat to get energy from plants. For all of human history, this has been the primary source of energy for the body.

Our primary question is "Why are we getting more diabetes and obesity over the last generation or so?" I am contending most of this is related to our diet. Then, of course, the next question is "What is it in our diet that is causing this?" That's what I'm trying to explain to you right now. Later it will be "What can I do about it?" We will get to that at the end.

First, starch in its natural form may not digest very well at all. Cooking markedly increases digestibility and hence the energy recovery from starch. I am not sure when man began cooking meals, but it was probably close to the beginning of human history. Historical man was pretty smart. We know that a little increase in cortisol enhances memory and thinking. Nothing jacks up you cortisol a little like not having a supermarket around or wondering if there is a bear in the woods or looking for that next Viking invasion. Also, if you were smart, you probably increased your chance of survival. If not, no kids for you. Therefore, I am going to assume the cooking of starch has been around most of the time.

Unlike sucrose, even cooked starch has a complicated path to digestion and hence glucose absorption. It also needs water molecules, and a few extra enzymes. Although starch is a string of glucose molecules, it is initially digested into the disaccharide maltose, a molecule of two glucose molecules. Then this is further digested into glucose, then absorbed with all the other glucose molecules. As you can see, it is not quite as available as sucrose, but we can still speed it up.

Most starch has some nondigestible starch in it called fiber. It is also composed of glucose, but humans do not have the enzyme to separate these particular glucose-to-glucose bonds, so it passes through the small intestine. We will get a little energy out of it later.

This intermixed fiber slows down digestion as it makes it more difficult for the enzymes (amylases) to get to the starch molecules and convert them eventually to glucose. You can see the same process in fruits and fructose. The fiber in fruit slows down the digestibility of the sugars and delays and spreads out the absorption. Of course, you bypass this when you eat just the juice, and we are back to drinking sugar water.

We cook starches and that greatly improves digestibility and glucose absorption. For most humans, grains have been the primary source of starch and hence energy. If we look at grains as opposed to root vegetables, we see that we also have that fiber intermixed in the starch. To remind you, grain has the bran which is non-digestible starch(fiber), the endosperm which is starch, and the germ which is protein and fat (and the vitamins). Throughout history, the main starch has been some type of wheat or rice. Nowadays, corn also provides a significant amount of starch (and glucose). If you just ate them raw, you would get very little nutrition. You need to remove the outer husk to let your digestive enzymes get access to the nutrients inside. I imagine at the beginning of human history, they ate the whole grain and got what nutrition they could by chewing the husk to get to the germ, but after about a week or two they decided there must be a better way and milling was developed.

Milling is the process of crushing the grain particles so as you can separate the bran from the endosperm and hence get access to the starch energy. In the beginning, the entire grain, including the bran, was used to make bread. Bread making seems to have existed at the beginning, and this was the most common way to consume wheat.

Almost all the same can be said for rice grain, but this was not made into bread.

The wheat grain contains the protein gluten which enables us to make bread. The grain must be crushed to a certain minimum size to make bread, and this size remained consistent for thousands of years. The bran was eventually separated from the crushed grain to give a better color to the bread and enable a less dense product. As time went on, the germ was also separated, and we have what we have today. Today whole wheat bread means you separate the components, then add it back to make whole wheat flour.

Let me review my conundrum. I believe the basis for our obesity problem revolves around insulin resistance. I believe this occurs by repeated exposure to glucose spikes over the years. Carbohydrates drive insulin secretion. The easy mark is sucrose. This has been more readily available in the last hundred years, has been processed into much of our food, and has increased with our current intake of soda pop. I compare this with history, in which obesity and diabetes have not been a problem. It is not hard to conclude that a high carb diet may be the basis for the current problem. But I just can't blame it all on sugar. The consumption by the United States has been dropping, and as I mentioned, much of our carbohydrate intake is from starch, not sugar.

So maybe we are just eating too much bread and pasta. This increased with the government advocating a low-fat diet, which you know by now means a high carbohydrate diet. The adoption of this concept may well be a major contributor to our current problems. Still, I can't get around the observation that a somewhat high carbohydrate diet has been present throughout history. The carbohydrates have come mainly from grains in the form of wheat and rice. Both must be milled somewhat to get access to the nutrients. Bread has been the method, in the western world, for which I have the most written records, by which these carbohydrates were consumed. It doesn't make sense for me to blame bread for our problems: or does it?

Around 1850-1900, there were several reports in which explorers interacted with cultures that were independent of Western society. This varied between Inuit people, isolated western Pacific islands, Indians in the southwest of America, or much of the southern continent of Africa. The British especially had detailed records of their hospitals in Africa. Upon interaction with these cultures, western culture and diet were introduced. The previous diet varied from a high carb, very low carb, and balanced. These cultures had previously survived and prospered on their local diet for thousands of years.

We provided these cultures with food, and at that time the preserved food was biscuits (bread), molasses (sucrose), and salted meats. Invariable, these populations began to develop Western diseases such as diabetes and obesity. Several medical missionary reports showed that modern diseases in these cultures did not exist until the adoption of a Western-type diet. No, don't get me wrong. Civilization improved the overall lifespan with modern sanitation and the prevention of destructive cultural practices, but we may have just extended the lifespan, not the healthy lifespan.

So why did this happen? Some of these cultures on the Pacific islands had a high carb diet. With the introduction of the Western diet, we may not have raised their carbohydrate intake at all. Yet there appeared to be something different about the Western diet that lead them down the road to Western disease. I have already talked about sucrose, and these cultures may well have gone from virtually no sucrose related carbs to a good portion. Remember, if there are sweet things around, man likes to eat it: but right now, I am going to talk about flour.

Grain was milled thousands of years. Initially, it was done by hand, and still is in some places. Man was smart enough to develop stone wheels that could be ground together to crush the grain to a fairly small size, maybe 500 microns. This ended up being a good size grain to be able to make decent bread and, although dark and dense, it served its purpose. To review, grain has protein and starch. The protein is somewhat elastic allowing us to add yeast to produce carbon dioxide. The elastic protein can contain this gas so that the bread rises, and you have a less dense bread which is more desirable. If you take out the bran, you get an even less dense bread which is lighter in color. We have done this in some form for the last few thousand years.

With the onset of the industrial revolution, we figured out how to use steam to turn these wheels and production of flour increased. Eventually, we skipped the stone wheels and went to steel rollers. Driven by capitalism, we made these flour grains smaller and smaller. As the resulting bread had a better texture and would sell better.

We now can crush particles to a size smaller than red blood cells. Now we don't do that to the flour we buy in the store, but I believe we are at a size that is much smaller than what man ate historically. Look carefully at your flour. Are you able to even see one grain (maybe if you are young and have good eyesight), but it is much smaller than just a couple hundred years ago?

Go back to sucrose. Grain is starch. Starch is glucose. Starch must be broken down to glucose just like sucrose, except now we are getting 100% glucose. As I mentioned earlier, starch is a little more complicated and takes a little more time to metabolize, but like sucrose, as the particles get smaller the enzymes have better access to the surface area. The surface area to volume ratio increases dramatically with smaller size particles. I believe this may explain how man could eat bread for thousands of years without developing obesity in a large proportion of the population. Similarly, giving flour to indigenous populations increased obesity, even though you may not have increased their carb intake significantly.

I'll talk more about grain at the end of the book (if I remember), but the short version is that the grain itself may have changed slightly, but the processing has changed a lot, especially over the last hundred years. Even with the small particle size it probably doesn't give that big spike with sucrose, which is getting close to IV (intravenous) glucose, but it does decrease the time it takes to make flour glucose available for absorption. I believe shortens the time for glucose absorption and insulin secretion leading to an overall more rapid rise in insulin than we have had in times past.

Carbohydrates drive insulin. The more rapidly you absorb glucose, the more rapidly the insulin level rises. The area under the curve may be about the same, but it is shifted to the left with rapid absorption vs a slow absorption over a longer time.

I will repeat, I believe insulin resistance is primarily a result of multiple exposures to elevated insulin levels. I believe this is exacerbated if the spikes are higher and more numerous. This problem has gotten worse in modern times so that now we have a 40% obesity rate, something not seen in the history of man. I believe diet is the primary culprit in driving this disease. I believe carbohydrates in the diet are the key. I believe the carbohydrates in modern man's diet are not the same as historical man, mainly due to processing, and is the main factor in the development of insulin resistance. It probably is not only the total amount but also the composition. Carbohydrates drive insulin and abnormal insulin secretion drives insulin resistance.

Food Engineer

I started with the observation that modern man is getting fat and getting type two diabetes. Both are a reflection of insulin resistance, whereby it takes a slightly higher level of insulin to get the blood sugar down to a certain set point. This begins a cascade of greater fat storage, more hunger, more frequent intake of food, decreased autophagy, increased epigenetic changes in DNA, changes in gut biome, increased stimulation of the immune system, higher levels of autoimmune disease, and decreased overall health. It is a cumulation of 20 – 40 years of diet, not a week of partying at a resort.

I have concentrated my efforts to explain this obesity epidemic by the effects of diet. I think this is the major factor, but realize that the environment, with our exposure to chemicals not seen in a natural state, contribute to some of our ills. I also believe in a progressive deterioration of the human genome and epigenome that slowly affects mankind. But diet is a condition that we can change in our life here and now. Although all of my diet books can stand alone on the topic addressed in each one, the basic theme is how did we get to our current levels of obesity and what can be do about it? What particularly in our diet should we change? How does our diet affect other aspects of our health? What foods should we be buying and eating? How often should we eat and not eat?

This book is a continuation of the book *Maintenance Diet for the Modern Man*. That book talked about protein, fat, and carbohydrates in the diet and gave recommendations about what to do with them in our diet. I emphasized the role of the food engineer. This person must purchase the food. There usually is not an unlimited budget and assessing the value of the dollar spent is a slowly acquired skill. Now they must determine how much food to buy based upon demand and storage capacity. There must be thoughts involved as to what the menu is to be. Not only today but throughout the week. Each menu may have particular requirements for its preparation. There is the actual examination of the food bought. What has been added by the producer in the way of additional chemicals to ensure freshness and preservation? Where did the food come from? How were the animals fed? Do we have to worry about chemicals applied to fresh foods? Does it need to be whole grain or is processed grain OK? How much processing can we live with?

Finally, the food engineer has left the store. Now home to begin preparation. Are there any special requirements for the family, after all, they may be preparing for people with various calorie or nutritional requirements. It may be wise to give a five-year-old whole milk, but not a sixty -year- old. Then how much food to prepare? If food supplies were adequate, through much of history people ate till they were not hungry, then stopped. Estimating food amounts is an acquired skill. Don't forget there are mealtimes. The food engineer must have everything ready at certain agreed-upon times such that everyone can show up and eat. Timing the preparation is in itself a separate skill. In many families, the engineer must prepare to-go meals that have their own special requirements. In many families with young kids and teenagers, there may be an additional requirement to have snack material available. In all my books I have encouraged the concept of not eating for 12 hours between the first and last meal. Now the engineer must cram all the eating into a 12 -hour window. Of course, the family assumes food safety, that is the food has been prepared appropriately and stored to avoid bacterial growth.

For most of history, it was the wife of the husband who assumed this role. You can see, this is a full-time job, although the wife also had many other responsibilities in maintaining the home. The diminishing of the role as a homemaker has paralleled the expansion of the diagnosis of obesity. Many now have a job outside the family. They simply do not have enough time to devote their efforts to the family diet. Shortcuts must be made like eating out more, buying already prepared foods and snacks, preferring convenience over preparation, or using fast-food restaurants to rapidly fill in meals for the family. There is no doubt this contributes to a diet that may encourage insulin resistance, a diet foreign to most of mankind's existence.

In today's world, it is quite possible to eat out every meal and bypass the food engineer. The restaurant's food engineer can provide you enough food to satisfy any appetite, at almost any hour of the day whenever you show up. But the goal is not a diet for health, it is to provide a service to earn a living. In my lifetime, eating out once or twice a month was considered to be an event. Now every family may eat out at a restaurant, at a fast-food place, at the grocery store, or the convenience store almost every day. Eating pre-prepared food is eating out. Virtually all of the products will contribute to insulin resistance.

The food engineer gets the honor, but also the blame. For the most part, she has control over what the family eats. If the family is overweight, the food engineer is responsible. Your kids eventually leave home, but if the food engineer has done her job, they will usually continue to eat well. If your 14-year-old is fat, I'm afraid it is probably the diet you are providing. If your husband is fat, it may be the diet you are providing. You are the food expert, and I am trying to give you the knowledge you need to make a reasonable decision that can avoid obesity and eventual insulin resistance.

Significance of Bread in Human History

I started this book as an addendum to the previous book. If you remember my conundrum, I believe a lower carb diet to be a defense against obesity. Bread is a high carb item. Why then does bread play such a prominent role in man's history, but obesity does not. The more I studied and thought about this subject, the more elevated the status of bread in history became clearer. I have used the Bible as a historical source for diet. I can apply this to the history of bread in the history of man.

The first mention of bread is at the expulsion of Adam:

Gen 3:19, In the sweat of thy face shalt thou eat bread, till thou return unto the ground;

From the beginning, bread was eaten. This is the oldest processed food. Indications are that bread was a major part of the diet. For the next 1500 years, no meat was eaten in the diet (although animal products were used). The nutrition from bread and other plant products enabled man to thrive and expand. Although the exact grain cannot be ascertained, we do know that the Nile River Valley soon became the principal grower of wheat in the world. We are pretty sure that Emmer wheat was the primary grain. Bread was then mentioned over 200 times in the Old Testament over a period covering 4000 years. It was often mentioned as the primary source of nutrition and often mentioned as the only food given. Of particular interest is the seven-year Egyptian famine. Prior to the famine, there were seven years of plenty during which time excess grain was stored. During the famine, the grain was sold to the surrounding countries. People traveled to get grain so that they could live. The only food for a large portion of the population was bread made from grain. This is historically significant in that history indicates bread was the primary means of preventing starvation. It also implies that all that was required to survive would be bread and water. As we have seen from examining whole wheat flour, it may be that bread alone could keep you alive through periods of starvation. As I have mentioned, grain has been the principal food that man could store for times of scarcity, and perhaps this was sufficient to avoid starvation. This is even reflected in the New Testament with the metaphor Jesus used:

Matt 4:3-4, And when the tempter came to him, he said. If thou be the Son of God, command that these stones be made bread.

But he answered and said, It is written. Man shall not live by bread alone, but by every word that proceedeth out of the mouth of God

This supports the numerous references and implications that for thousands of years, bread alone could be eaten to maintain life, especially in times of scarcity when starvation was a possibility.

A modern-day reflection of this can be seen in the Green Revolution which took place during the 1950s – 1960s. This was personified in Norman Borlaug, who led the development of a dwarf, disease resistant, high yielding wheat grains that markedly increased grain production throughout the world and virtually eliminated starvation in many countries. Providing food security resulted in his being presented with the Nobel Peace Prize, the Presidential Medal of Freedom, and the Congressional Gold Medal. It also again demonstrated the power of bread to relieve starvation.

Bread changed little for thousands of years. It was whole wheat and stone ground. There were no additives. This bread was dense, hard and not that easy to eat; yet it was embraced by mankind as an answer to starvation. That's not to say that given the opportunity, man ate all kinds of other things; but bread remained the cornerstone for a sustained diet. Despite the high carbohydrate load, bread eating did not appear to produce a lot of insulin resistance. Now, you recognize that bread today is not the same as bread a few hundred years ago.

I have tried to replicate modern bread using large particle grinding of whole wheat flour and cannot even come close. The bread I make is hard and somewhat difficult to eat, although it is tasty. I looked through the pastry, cake, and roll section of my local grocery store. There was no whole wheat. All were composed of highly processed, finely ground, white flour. None would have been available a few hundred years ago. The bread section was quite similar, although I could find a few with whole wheat and stone ground. Still, this bread looked nothing like the bread I could make, nor like that eaten for most of history.

Modern bread has about the same number of carbohydrates as historical bread, but the nutritional content has been reduced and processing has changed the way it is absorbed by your body, changed the amount of nutrition you obtain, and probably changes your gut biome. It contains chemicals never used before in bread up to recent times. There is no doubt the modern world has an epidemic of obesity/diabetes/insulin resistance. I have no doubt that the modern diet is driving insulin resistance. Our modern food has been processed such that it leads to more rapid, more frequent, and higher elevations of insulin in response to elevated levels of glucose. The increased consumption of carbohydrates in our diet in response to government diet recommendations, modern belief in the danger of fats and proteins, production of more flavorful foods, and modern advertising have all markedly contributed to this process. Now the historical basis for our diet, that is bread, has been perverted to the point that I am not sure you could survive on a diet of modern bread and water. Even modern economics, which has led to the diminution of the food engineer to someone who figures out where were go out to eat today, has added to this epidemic. We have plenty of food, plenty of money, and get plenty of exercise, but that is not keeping us from getting fat. It is difficult to control your exposure to environmental toxins, but you can control your diet.

We can't get around the fact that the wheat we use today is not the same as the wheat used thousands of years ago. As I discussed previously, grain has been cross bred throughout human history and hundreds of thousands of crossbreds have been made. We are pretty sure that Emmer was used by the Egyptians, but there are species (Einhorn) that existed prior to that time. Most wheat varieties now are some form of the dwarf type. The nutrient profile is different from the profiles of the most common varieties fifty years earlier. These probably had a slightly different nutritional profile than those a few hundred years earlier. That's not to say it is better or worse, but it is different.

In addition, the nutritional qualities of the grain vary depending on what region of the country it was grown, and even on what farm it was grown. The micronutrients can change with what fertilizer (if any) was used, was the land allowed to lay fallow, were nitrogen-fixing crops grown on the land, and how long the land has been under cultivation. It would be very difficult for us to determine these variables, whether buying grain, flour, or bread. I advise we look at the variables we can actually control. The type of wheat is sometimes known, especially when buying grain or flour. Unfortunately, right now I don't know what to recommend. We have control if we are buying whole wheat flour or bread. Remember, roller milling means we have removed the bran and germ, ground the endosperm to a smaller particle size, then add back the other elements. We can pretty much be sure that if the grain was stone ground and the first pass was used, the particle size would be larger than almost all modern flour and bread. There are various additives to flour to enable modern machinery to turn out perfect loaves of bread that have little rising time but have been created to form the correct crumb structure, mouthfeel, soft texture, and long shelf life. No considerations have been made to nutrition except the enrichment with a few artificial vitamins and minerals.

Few of you will cook your own bread. If you do, you have a great variety of flour you can buy online.

Hardly anyone will grind their own flour, but those that do have control over what they get.

Finally, you can buy sourdough bread. Almost all will have a smaller particle size.

You can make your own sourdough, and you can make it with whatever flour you want. But as we have discovered, it is difficult to make light fluffy bread using large particle whole wheat flour.

I hate to say it as this will defeat the purpose of the book, but you could just not eat bread. With the advent of the low carb diet, many people do not eat bread. Also, no cake, rolls, cupcakes, donuts, or any pastry. People do this every day if you are on a low carb maintenance diet. For those who have been diagnosed with prediabetes/Type 2 diabetes or those with insulin resistance and subsequent obesity, you will be counting your carbs. Therefore, you will be going light on the bread, regardless of what kind of bread. In the modern diet, you are not reliant on bread to provide you with basic proteins and nutrients. You have many other options available as to what to eat, and there is lots of food around. A thousand years ago you may have had to eat bread or die. People with celiac are used to avoiding wheat bread all their life.

This book is an addendum to *Maintenance Diet for the Modern Man*. For a normal, lifetime diet, I do not advise a low carb diet. I do advise a diet lower than 50% total carbohydrates, because I believe the food has changed and hence, we cannot go back to the historical higher carb diet. Therefore, I do not advise total abstinence from bread: but if you eat bread, I advise you to choose wisely using the information I have provided in this book.

Wrap up

The more glucose, the more insulin. The more often, the more frequent are these insulin spikes. Do this 7 times a day for 30 years and you have about 80,00 insulin spikes. Only takes a little increase in the normal spike and you get insulin resistance. Of course, you don't have to eat seven times a day, and you don't always have to get the maximum spike. Depends on your diet.

Sucrose in water is basically IV (intravenous) glucose and is rapidly absorbed and quickly raises the insulin spike. Frequently exposing the gut to glucose gives you many spikes of insulin and an increased total volume under the curve of insulin production.

Fiber in grain (and fruit) comes in two forms, soluble and insoluble. The insoluble passes through the gut and can be digested in the lower parts of the intestine by bacteria to provide energy, nutritional chemicals, and vitamins. Insoluble fiber forms a gel in the stomach and prolongs digestion as the enzymes cannot get to the food particles as rapidly. This is why eating whole fruit does not give you as rapid a glucose spike as fruit juice. It is also why starch in root vegetables and whole-grain delays somewhat the absorption of glucose, and hence you do not get as high an insulin peak. Although the total absorbed glucose may be the same (or less), the insulin peak isn't as high. Making food particles smaller increases access to digestive enzymes and promotes more rapid and complete absorption. The overall effect is to increase the speed and amount of glucose absorption.

If you are in a starvation mode, you want all the glucose you can get. It appears a high carb diet does not lead to obesity if you are low on food. If you are not in a starvation mode, rapid absorption does eventually lead to insulin resistance, especially if you are eating often.

Modern bread making has not only eliminated much of the soluble fiber in bread by removing the bran, but also diminished the particle size of the flour. Your body seems to have been created such that larger particle size and fiber protects against the eventual development of insulin resistance, despite a large carbohydrate load. The balance seems to be somewhat delicate as cutting the average particle size in half and eliminating most of the fiber is enough to induce this condition. This may be why eating stone-ground whole grain for thousands of years did not lead to insulin resistance.

We have been eating bread for the history of man and will probably continue to do so. It is possible in our modern world to go without eating wheat bread at all, but requires a little work, and I don't know that would be the healthiest diet. We would have to ignore dietary history. Nevertheless, there is a small number of people who simply cannot tolerate wheat well. My recommendations for the lifelong maintenance diet are:

Particle size drives absorption. Bread made from stone ground flour will give you a large size distribution hence slow down rapid uptake. If the whole wheat bread is white and fluffy, something has been added to make it that way or the flour has been milled to decrease particle size. If it says 100% whole wheat, it probably has not been roller milled. Then look at the ingredient list. I have found that you really cannot make softer bread with larger particles flour without adding extra gluten. Go organic.

If you make your own bread (and I recommend this), buy stone-ground whole-wheat flour. I recommend using a sour dough starter. You may need extra gluten (Vital Wheat Gluten)

For pasta, look at the ingredients. Use those with only semolina used as the ingredient. This will be Durham wheat. This will almost always mean larger particles unless they have also added Durham flour. Whole wheat if you can. Maybe use this instead of bread. It has the same number of carbs.

For those few of you who grind your own wheat, a fine grind on most machines will give you a good particle size distribution. For Vitamix, four cups of grain, high speed thirty seconds, shake, repeat three times for total of 2 minutes. You shake to prevent insure even distribution and to give the flour a chance to cool down a little.

Pastry requires fine flour and is not whole wheat. I can't really make them healthy, but a lifetime maintenance diet requires deserts. Use you common sense and don't eat them all the time or on an empty stomach.

Do not forget oats. They are not ground into flour, simply crushed. It has virtually no additives, has lots of soluble fiber which mutes the insulin surge, has many valuable nutrients, and is about the least processed food you can get. Unfortunately, they have a somewhat dull taste, so you often add something to them. Don't just cover them with sugar. Buy organic oats if possible as some oats may have Roundup residue.

A few of you cannot eat whole wheat flour secondary to reactions to proteins found in the bran and germ. Use organic, white bread flour with as few additives as possible. Make sure you go sour dough if you can. See addendum on WGA.

This book deals with only a part of the maintenance diet and is an extension of Maintenance *Diet for the Modern Man.* Grains have been eaten forever and are a part of this diet. Although I encourage as little processing as possible, grains need to have a little to get rid of the antinutrients present and perhaps harmful proteins. They need to be ground to access the nutrients. Water and heat are required to access the starch well. Fermentation with yeast and lactic acid bacteria (sourdough) breaks down many of the harmful proteins in the grain as well as making the final product more palpable.

Grains contain proteins that may be harmful to us. Your intestinal barrier can often keep these from being absorbed, and hence, man has been able to eat bread for thousands of years without difficulty. In the modern world, our gut microbiome has been changed for the worse which affects the intestinal barrier and may make us more susceptible to eating grains. This is not the historical state of man.

The gut microbiome is a complex subject and requires its own book. This book helps the food engineer construct the maintenance diet.

Wheat germ agglutinin

Lectins are a group of proteins that bind to carbohydrates and are present in plants. These serve as defensive elements against external pathogens such as bacteria, fungi, and insects. The most common lectin we hear about in bread is gluten and we have seen that this can adversely affect some individuals by interacting with their immune system. Lectins are routinely used in scientific testing to bind to various glycoproteins, and we eat lectins every day in our normal diet.

Of interest in nutrition is a lectin called wheat germ agglutinin (WGA), found in cereal wheat germ. WGA has been accused of having adverse health effects both by binding to cells in the gut and causing damage, and by being absorbed into the body and having direct effects on various cells as well as the immune system. As a result, some have advised us to avoid whole wheat bread as normal flour bread has had the bran and germ removed, thus lowering the amount of WGA exposure.

WGA may be able to replicate some of the actions of insulin, such as encouraging fat cells to absorb glucose and turn it into fat, thus promoting obesity. Various effects of WGA on cells can be demonstrated in cells in the laboratory.

Let's look a little more closely. In a recent thesis (Kuzma, 2009), consumption of 50 grams of wheat germ, the equivalent of eating 80 slices of whole wheat bread, was given to normal people. Blood samples were taken regularly up to 24 hours later and no WGA was detected. It may be the level was lower than the sensitivity of the tests, but certainly a large amount was not absorbed.

It can also be shown that heat treatment (cooking) greatly affects the biological activity of dietary lectin WGA. We already process grains with yeast and bacteria to enhance absorption of nutrients, and these processes may also diminish the WGA burden.

We can show in animals that a high WGA intake can adversely affect the gut microbiome and affect inflammatory markers and white blood cells.

Some believe that dietary lectin uptake can affect wight gain by causing leptin resistance, a hormone that signals the brain to stop eating and hence could trigger over-eating. All these affects are shown in cell cultures or possibly animals, but no definitive studies in humans.

On the other hand, there have been studies showing that whole grain consumption is associated with a lower BMI. There have been human studies that show the consumption of whole grain is related to improved blood glucose control. Regular consumption of whole grain products is associated with a significant reduction of the risk of Type 2 diabetes, heart disease, and weight gain.

The human body is amazingly complex. When I see no definitive support for a dietary recommendation, I conclude we may just not understand what is going on.

There are some people who seem to have an intolerance to wheat, but don't have celiac disease or wheat allergy. It may be that these people may be better able to tolerate wheat flour in which the bran and germ have been removed and the flour bleached, all which will lower the WGA. These people may be able to tolerate white bread without difficulty and, if so, should avoid whole wheat bread. I don't know if this is a WGA issue or something else; it doesn't really matter to the food engineer; she just adjusts the maintenance diet appropriately.

We have been eating whole wheat bread from the beginning. I know something has changed over the last 100 years leading us to obesity. Food processing has changed as has wheat genetics. Right now, I am sticking with my whole wheat bread, stone ground or at least large particle size, organic, and sourdough starter. It has been this way a long time and I will need better evidence to change my recommendation. I agree there are a few who should not eat gluten, and probably a few who should not eat whole wheat; but for most of us, I still believe this is the right way to go.

As I proceed through writing my books on diet and health, I can't help but get the impression that the gut microbiome and corresponding intestinal barrier may be the basis for many of these nutritional and immunological dysfunctions. The modern diet and environment are affecting us in many ways. I am trying to get you to change the things over which you have control to achieve better health, not to make you live forever.

PARTICLE SIZE

I have talked about particle size, now for some numbers. The traditional stone milled flour as always been screened in some manner, as too large of a particle adversely affects the texture. This is usually done with a 40-mesh screen which prevents particles larger than 420 microns from entering the flour. This is also the screen used in semolina flour; thus, all the particles are less than this size. In modern flour, the average size of the particle is about 120 microns, although some are finer.

I have experimented with the particle size and found that no matter what I do to the dough, I cannot get a good rise if more than about 10% of the flour particles are larger than 420 microns. In commercial whole wheat mills this is about the percentage of particles greater than 420.

The next dividing line is 250 microns (60-mesh) Sieving the flour gives about 35-60 percent of the particles above this size. The remaining particles are less than this size. As near as I can tell, this was about the size flour particles that were used the last few thousand years. Remember, if you keep running the flour through the mill again, you will increase the amount of fine flour. This was certainly done in the past and the fine flour was special. Most of the time the first pass was used.

I experimented with my Vitamix and could get this approximate range of particle size with the two-minute 30 second grind on high (four cups of grain). I used a commercial home grinder and the fine setting also gave me a similar result.

I experimented baking loaves of bread (I only used two cup loaves as I was just interested in the rise and texture) and was able to get a decent rise using sourdough starter. You must let it rest awhile before baking. Using store bought yeast instead of sourdough I got a slightly better rise and did not have to let it rest as long. I could get a better rise on both if I added a little extra gluten (vital wheat gluten)

It appeared that I had to get to the stone-ground particle size to get a decent rise. Anything larger left me with a dense bread that was somewhat difficult to eat (or even cut)

Using all-purpose flour (which is entirely less than 250 microns) made it much easier to get a rise and it simulated store-bought bread. Commercial bread has many other additives to make it light and fluffy (and increase the shelf life): This has been the goal of bakers for hundreds of years.

As you must know by now, I do not believe eating white fluffy is worth it. Traditional stone-ground bread milled to at least the size I have mentioned gives you good tasting edible bread. Any larger, the bread is not very palpable. Much smaller and you get light and fluffy, but also perhaps an increased risk of obesity and diabetes. If you must buy bread, get 100% whole wheat. It is difficult to buy 100% whole wheat sourdough bread since you need a small particle size to get a fluffy good rise. I had to add a little gluten to my sourdough to get a good rise.

As I have mentioned, obesity may be related to your gut microbiome, and the many additives of store bought white fluffy bread may be adversely affecting this biome.

I have taught you enough to at least understand the ingredient list and make as wise a decision as you can.

More books by this author:

Diet and Health

Diabetes, Prediabetes Obesity

Ketogenic Diet for Beginners

Fasting and Autophagy

Maintenance Diet

Bread In the Modern Diet

Epigenetics In Pregnancy

Introduction to Cell Biology and Epigenetics

Diet and Disaster: Food Shortage

Covid and Vaccines for Medical Professionals
Covid and Vaccines for the Common Man
Allulose and Other Sweeteners
Practical Sex for Older Married Couples
Sexuality in Marriage After Fifty
eBook A2 Milk
eBook Brain Disease and Fasting
eBook Tampons and Cancer
eBook Let's Rename PCOS
eBook Weight Loss for Women
eBook-Fat Kids and Fasting
eBook Lipoproteins in Diet and Health
eBook Autophagy and Ages
eBook Carbs for Food Engineers
eBook Fructose and Soy for Food Engineers
eBook Fasting and Disease
eBook Know Your Orgasm
(for advertising Know Your Organ)
eBook Know Your Masturbation
eBook Know Your Clitoris
(for advertising Know Yourself)
eBook Artificial Sweeteners and the Gut Biome
eBook 28 Day Fast
eBook Dementia in Women
eBook Fat and Protein for Food Engineers
eBook The Food Engineer
eBook Flour Treatment
eBook Bread Gluten and Sensitivity
eBook Introduction to Stem Cell
(Regenerative Cell) Treatment
eBook Prolonged Fasting
eBook Anorgasmia in Women